Healers,
Helpers,
Wizards
and
Guides:

A Healing Journey

Paul,
The world is a
bright happy place
with you in it!
Thank you!
Bertie

Bertie Ryan Synowiec, M.S.

Positive Support Seminars
and Publications
Grosse Ile, Michigan

Other books written by Bertie Ryan Synowiec:
- *Does Anyone Hear Our Cries For Help?*
- *Quick And Easy Self-Esteem Builders*
- *Ideario Constructivo De La Autoestima*
- *Affirmations For Increased Productivity*
- *Group Facilitation Handbook*
- *Teaching Students Strategies For Survival In A Dysfunctional Environment*
- *Success Strategies For A Positive Relationships I*
- *I'm A Pro At Hard Work*
- *Slow Isn't Bad. Fast Isn't Better. Different Isn't Wrong.*
- *Why Do You Force Me To Talk To A Chemical When All I Want Is Your Heart?*

Published by:

Positive Support Seminars and Publications
28641 Elbamar Drive, Grosse Ile, MI 48138-2013 U.S.A.
1-800-676-3806
http://www.bookzone.com/bookzone/10000641.html

Book and cover design:

Erkfitz & Associates, Riverview, MI

Healers, Helpers, Wizards and Guides: A Healing Journey
Copyright © 1999 by Bertie Ryan Synowiec, M.S.

Library of Congress Catalog Card Number: 99-90068

ISBN 1-885335-16-4: $14.95 Softcover

Printed in the United States of America

Table of Contents

About The Author

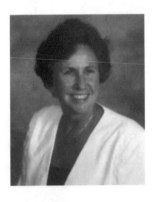

Bertie Ryan Synowiec, M.S., is a graduate of Wheeling Jesuit University in West Virginia and received her Masters Degree in Biology from Adelphi University in New York. A former Health Educator for twenty years and the mother of five children, she has also completed the course-work for a second Masters Degree in Educational Psychology. She is the author of ten books and has created a *Skill-Building System* that teaches individuals *Strategies for Successful Living in Dysfunctional Environments.*

Bertie is well known for her ability to clarify and en-hance the role of the individual in this ever changing world both at home and in the workplace. She is the founder and Director of Positive Support Seminars in Grosse Ile, Michigan and is an active member of the National Speakers Association. During her twelve years as a professional consultant, she has watched tremendous growth in individuals encour-aged through her programs, books and tapes to take respon-sibility for their own happiness with positive healthy choices that restore energy and motivation and create a wholeness in mindbodyspirit.

In Appreciation

I thank you – my healers, helpers, wizards and guides – for touching my life. You know who you are! Your spirit resides within the pages of this book and I acknowledge you with tremendous gratitude - My readers, reviewers, teachers, authors, editors, counselors, doctors, family and friends. With your everlasting encouragement, I trusted that this journey could be taken and I believed that it would all unfold exactly as it was meant to be.

With a quiet sense of humility, I thank my doctor for facilitating this healing process within me and for giving me a place of safety where I could be myself and reclaim my good health. I could not have taken this journey alone, and yet in his care, I was brought to a place of peaceful solitude.

I am also grateful to my husband, Dick, for his loving patience as he read and reread the script in its infancy and beyond and to my sisters, Teen, Pat and Barbara, for their endless wisdom and determination to make me clarify my thoughts over and over again. I also wish to thank our children, Rich, Laurie, Dan, Christy, Kevin, and daughter-in-law Beth, who "released me" with patience, love and understanding. "Mom, it's a best seller," our son told me. "Write it like a best seller!"

For each of you everyday in my heart I say a special prayer of thanksgiving to God for bringing you into my life and for helping me make this book happen!

Introduction

I sit here in my doctor's office looking into the eyes of my four month old grandchild. She is beautiful. Her world is secure and she is very loved. She giggles out loud and then laughs and smiles. Like her parents, grandparents and great grandparents, she is hypersensitive to her environment and responds to the energy around her. When it is tense, she is tense; when it is loving, she is at peace. She is perfect, created in the image and the likeness of God.

Today is my appointment with the Chiropractor. He is also going to check the alignment of the spine of the new baby. I lie face down on the adjustment table. Her mom places her face down on my back. The length of my right leg immediately changes. Through the energy field of my body, the baby's hip is adjusted by my doctor of chiropractic. My legs, again, become equal in length. I am in awe, encased in this bundle of love that rests quietly on my back.

Her mom takes her lovingly into her arms. As I stand, I pray that, somehow, she can always be protected from the pain that has created the need for me to experience this healing journey back to a time when, like this innocent child, I was truly myself.

Who we are does not depend on what other people think of us. When we live our lives through the eyes of others, co-dependent relationships are created that rob us of our self-esteem, our sense of purpose and our mission in life. In time, it can take us so far away from our true self that we no longer know who we are.

At times, as the healing mystery unfolded in its own time, I felt as if it were a never ending story. In the beginning it is filled with emerging wisdom and insights that finally make sense to me, as my awakening takes place in the final chapters.

I did not travel this journey alone, nor could it have happened without my commitment to the process. My doctor gave me something to believe in, me, as he facilitated the natural process of healing within my body. I did the work myself, as I walked through the pain. My wounds were deep and had to heal from the inside out.

I share it all with you in truth, unafraid of your judgment. You are my partner in this journey. I believe we are all connected. It has been a mindbodyspirit healing far beyond anything I ever thought possible. I am whole, balanced and strong again. I have let go so far that all that remains is my faith in God.

Healers, Helpers, Wizards and Guides: A Healing Journey contains powerful lessons learned through the guidance of those who come into our lives at just the right moment to help us heal and grow. These very special relationships touch our lives with wisdom and unconditional love. They give us the strength to reclaim our sense of purpose and mission in life and to better understand our path.

Personal injury, illness and the loss of loved ones affect change in each of us in a way that gives us a unique opportunity to rewrite the story of our lives. This book is about making time to take responsibility for our health and well being and at the same time, enjoying the results. It is a story of hope, love and encouragement that presents a personal challenge for those wishing to redirect their lives towards wholeness in mindbodyspirit.

Bertie Ryan Synowiec
Grosse Ile, Michigan

CHAPTER ONE

The Journey Begins

Quietly, I sat on the basement steps, my life suddenly moving in slow motion about to come to a full halt. My ankle was broken in two places. I heard it crack when I fell and landed on the stairs. My body had been desperately trying to tell me to slow down. I wanted to do this, but I was having tremendous difficulty knowing where to begin.

Was this broken leg God's way of telling me the time was now? What did this all mean? Why at this moment? Hadn't I been through enough? This was not what I had planned. It wasn't supposed to be this way.

For thirty years while raising five children, I certainly never had the time to break a leg. I was having great difficulty paying attention and listening in my busy world where reflection time was at a minimum. For good reasons I was caught up in a cycle of always doing and never just being.

Both of my ninety year old parents had recently died within three months of one another. I had just returned home from Long Island, after peacefully settling their estate. I also needed to finish the final stages of a high school graduation party for our last child and was getting ready for a summer wedding for our Navy son. Our "nest" was about to be empty and I really believed that it was time for me to get back to caring for my family of creation.

My story is a true story from the patient's side of a healing journey. My broken leg was only my wake-up call. A "simple" neck injury, several months later, brought me into Chiropractic care with a gifted Chiropractor who facilitated this healing process. Each of us must find our own facilitator – someone you can trust who provides a safe haven for you to be yourself. For me this was the beginning of a journey inward in mind, body and spirit that has given me opportunities for good health far beyond anything I ever thought possible – physically, emotionally and spiritually.

This all became very important to me. I was feeling immobilized without any sense of direction and much of my discomfort had become a normal part of my life. I also knew that I was off track and was no longer able to stay focused. I was looking for inner peace but had no idea how to get there.

Many times a major loss, illness or injury will trigger this confusion. In time we come to identify ourselves with this pain, fearful to move beyond it. As a health educator and seminar facilitator for many years, I often taught the lesson of detachment to others. Somehow, at this moment, caught up in all my own turmoil, I seemed to have forgotten everything.

I never felt like I had fallen into a negative cycle and could not get out. It was not that way at all. Things just happened in their own time and place and I accepted them as they came. I also had a willingness to accept the miracles in my life, as real.

What I did not know was the number of areas of healing in mind, body, and spirit that would take place.

In time I was to understand the difference between being healed and being cured. Not everyone is cured of an illness or injury, if the illness is defined as the absence of disease. We can choose to take the time to be healed, but not all things can be cured. I just wanted all the physical and emotional pain in my life to go away and I wanted it gone yesterday!

Sabotaging my own progress by giving up too soon, was not my intention. To stay with my commitment to "take care of me" was a big decision. It was my turn and I was going to take it and not allow myself to be compromised, like I had done so often in the past. Regaining my health became my first priority. I had run out of excuses for not doing this. I knew what I had to do to get it back. This became my personal challenge to allow the process of healing to take place within me.

With this decision I found myself working so hard to push myself past my fears that my co-dependency issues would return. I had kept silent for too many years. I was the quiet little sister; I was a dutiful daughter, wife and mother, who never moved out of the submissive child role until I woke up fifteen years ago and realized that I had a voice and my own purpose and mission in life.

Subconsciously this was all very familiar to me. I really believed cognitively that I had learned my lessons well over the last ten years. After all, I wrote the book, *Does Anyone Hear Our Cries For Help?* which deals with the issues of co-dependency, only to discover that no one was listening. If things in my life needed to be changed then I had to change them myself. I didn't want to have to learn those lessons again.

Yet, something was happening to my body and it was trying to explain itself in my mind. As a kinesthetic learner, I guess these lessons still needed to be worked out in my body. Chiropractic care was my way of doing just that, but little did I know how this would affect me.

My life was catching up with me. I had come to believe the myth that how I was feeling was just part of the aging process and normal for my age.

I later learned that it did not have to be this way. I did not have to feel old! I did not have to feel weak! I did not have to feel limited! I could take responsibility for my own health and give myself permission to ask the questions that would help me reclaim what I had lost along the way. There was a part of me that did not want to do the work. This was a resistance that I felt so strongly inside. I was physically and emotionally worn out.

Time is required to process the healing. I wanted to give myself permission to take that time.

I did not take this journey alone. Along the way I took the risk to share my story of what I was learning with others and asked for their support. Healers, helpers, wizards and guides are there for each of us as we open our hearts to them and accept their unconditional love, support and encouragement. They help us rethink our life story. Their task is to give to us that vision of hope.

Unknowingly, many of you have been a partner with me, as you reached out with your guidance, depending on where I was on any given day along my journey. This guidance was necessary to help me develop the coping skills necessary to understand the process of change.

I have become far richer and healthier because of your love, wisdom and understanding. Often without realizing your influence on me, you have affirmed my belief in the power of the healing relationship and the connection we all can have with one another. Without knowing it, you have helped me remain accountable for the positive health decisions I made for myself one day at a time along this path.

Janet Quinn, Ph.D., author of *Therapeutic Touch: A Home Study Course for Family Caregivers*, explains, "Being healed means that we have come to grips with our illness, or injury, and have accepted its place in our lives. From that place we can then watch the healing process unfold for its own good, unpredictably, in whichever way it chooses to go.

When we are most resistant, our body will still heal. It is the natural healing process within each of us, as human beings, that cannot be stopped. We do not have to be a believer for it to take place. It is just one of the wonderful mysteries of the human body."

I did not want to be a patient. I did not want to be accountable to anyone. I did not want to put in the time to get better, although for many reasons I had to make the time in order to heal physically and emotionally. I had so many questions and did not fully understand the process in which I had reluctantly agreed to participate.

The walls closed in on me. I began to revisit my feelings of entrapment that had sent me on a healing journey fifteen years ago to release me from my co-dependency issues.

This intensity awakened the analytical personality in me that sought cognitive information. I was literally driven to seek out the answers to the many questions that came to me. The books and tapes along with the glossary of terms listed in the back of this book were all part of that process.

I felt like I was back in school, but never at a desk. It took me a while to understand from where the true answers would come.

Exposure today to an extensive amount of medical information and an inherent belief that we need the expert to teach us, can create in us feelings of insecurity. This raises many questions that need to be addressed. When we listen to our body, we know and can trust that what we hear is true.

This can be our foundation. If we are to heal properly, we want to keep asking the right questions.

Sometimes we need to understand and accept that the individuals with the answers to those questions may not always want to take the time to listen. It is then that we let go of our expectations which only bring us frustration and go elsewhere to many different sources for the answers. We have been shut down for too long that often our silence has cost us our health.

> **People today are hungry for the right information presented in such a way that they can understand and use, as it applies to their own path in life.**

As inquisitive patients, clients and even friends, we are not necessarily asking for advice, but rather just gathering information. We are looking for someone, a healer, helper, wizard or guide with similar experiences, with whom we can share our thoughts and learn new attitudes and behaviors. This information can then be used to make informed decisions about our own health and well being.

God is also our internal guide. When things happen, we ask, "Why me, God? Why now? I have too many things to do. So many people need me right now." I had to learn to trust and to believe that everything I needed would come to me, as I let go of the things in my life that I could not control.

> **Our challenge is to reframe our attitude to believe that this illness or injury is not God punishing us. But rather, it is God redirecting us to review our life and to connect again with our purpose and mission. Often, it is our second chance to again learn one of life's lessons we did not get the first time!**

There are great rewards that come when you realize that it is your time to let others love you and care for you. This was a difficult challenge for me for I truly believed that I could do it all. I had spent a lifetime putting my own needs on the back burner in order to accommodate the needs of my parents, husband, children and students. I could give my love and attention to others, but for me to accept that same love and care in return was very difficult.

I did not like to ask anyone for help. My own co-dependent issues got in the way along with my training from childhood to rescue others, much more needy than me. Sometimes I just did not know how to respond to kindness, love and sincerity. John DeMartini in his wonderful book, *Count Your Blessings*, suggests that a simple "thank you" is the best answer. There is so much to be grateful for, if we only allow ourselves to see our world from that perspective. "One cannot be angry and grateful at the same time," he says so clearly.

As healers, helpers, wizards and guides for one another, we often choose to bring what we know to people who are not ready for our gift. We must be patient and realize that everything happens in its own time. Sometimes we serve only as a stepping stone in their journey along their path towards enlightenment. We are only the messengers who increase their awareness to their possible need for change. Their empowerment to act on this knowledge is what they must do for themselves.

I spent years not knowing any better, or even just knowing, but not acting on this knowledge. This time, when the teacher appeared, the student was ready. No one else can do this for us. These are choices we make for ourselves, as we believe we deserve them. They have not always been easy!

With every new experience I believed that there was a message for me somewhere and that my personal challenge was to discover the lesson.

Very often we have difficulty understanding the element of time required for healing to take place. I knew this and chose to take that time. The thought of not succeeding never occurred to me. I learned to trust my instincts and listen to my body and allow myself to heal. It was not an easy task.

The following guidelines helped give me permission to believe I could do this:
- Right where I am is where I am supposed to be.
- All I get done in a day is all I'm supposed to do.
- Everything happens in its right time.
- All that I need in life will be given to me
- Sometimes all we can do is love others exactly as they are.
- I can let go again and again and again until I get it.

This has been a time for me to give back to myself at least as much time as I have so willingly given to others in my life. Others around me might not understand my choice to take care of me. That was going to be all right. As long as I understood and acted out of integrity, then I did not need approval. I used healthy detachment skills that I have worked on for years. This prevented me from internalizing the judgments and opinions of others who might not approve or understand what I needed.

Who I am and what I am choosing to do did not require the approval of anyone. It was my time and that time was now. It was also time to allow me this freedom.

This whole experience forced me to look at everything I knew from a different perspective. I had to rethink my priorities and remember who I was and why I do what I do and get back to being me. This realization and my determination to trust the healing process, helped create the many positive and wonderful changes in my life.

The following stories contain much hope in the fulfillment of those things in our lives that turn out to be our greatest opportunity to learn some powerful lessons. When I began this process I was making healthy decisions based on my gut feelings and instincts. Once these were set into motion, there was no turning back. I paid attention to my internal signals and began to heal, as I consciously became my own healer.

Today I feel fifteen years younger and ten pounds lighter than I ever felt when I began this healing journey. Emotionally, I am off the roller coaster. I no longer feel overwhelmed as if carrying the weight of a hundred years of inherited baggage on my shoulders. I also now require two hours less sleep a night than I have ever needed before!

CHAPTER TWO

Stepping Off The Fast Track…Abruptly

The day I broke my leg I learned a lot about the influence and power of the mind in healing process. Once I got past the initial shock, I was actually laughing. The ankle was turned in a way that legs don't move. "Pay backs are good," I said to my son, as he carried me to the car to take me to the emergency room. Who knows how many times I had done that for him in his lifetime? Four hours later I still felt no pain. He would answer, "Just you wait!" My injury required surgery to put in some pins and a steel plate for support, but that could not be done for about eight hours, when the doctor would be available.

Finally, after five hours the ankle was becoming a bit sensitive, but manageable. They offered me a pain killer. Not knowing any better and only following directions from those whom I believed knew more than me, I took it.

Within a moment the medication literally wiped away all my natural endorphins that I had built up with all my laughter. They were there, created by my body to protect me from the pain of my broken leg. It was like clearing a slate clean. I watched it happen, as if I was looking from the inside out.

With one quick sweep the pain took over — constant pain, not in intervals, like when you are having a baby. My blood pressure had dropped severely and they could give me nothing else. My husband felt so helpless and all we could do is watch the clock and wait out the next four hours.

I had no way of knowing that when we take certain prescription drugs their effects override the natural defenses of the body to heal. As these medications cover up the symptoms and we are still left with the cause, we find ourselves recovering more from the side effects of the medicine than from the illness or injury. The pain killer did not even touch the problem.

I had been really doing fine without it for the time being, but I forgot to ask about my options. It was my job to ask, not theirs! They were just doing what they always have done and that was to give the patient some medication.

With an hour remaining they offered me morphine. I knew enough about my own addictive personality and the fact that my sister had difficulty in surgery with that drug affecting her blood pressure, that I chose not to take it.

The hour remaining before surgery was probably one of the longest hours in my life. I thought of my brother-in-law, a doctor and dear friend and asked my husband to call him from my room. He would know what was going on with me and would also take my mind off the pain of my broken leg. He understood my premed background from college and with textbook accuracy began to medically describe how morphine affects the body and why the blood pressure drops and what structural components go where and do what.

I was fascinated and honored to have such a healer and guide in my life. His connection with me took care of my need for the morphine and the hour passed.

He was a Godsend and had always been there for all of his own children and nieces and nephews. We had our own private pediatrician through the years who made "house calls" at our family gatherings.

Having been on the fast track for a lifetime, I was really ready for a vacation - even if it was one at home with a full cast on my leg. Where other couples had two children, we had five. When I was thirty-five years old, my world was falling apart from exhaustion. I figured I had lived many years in double time, so that, if something had happened to me then, I was really double my age and had led a full life.

When I found the following poem, I wondered, if it was written specifically for me.

Slow Me Down, Lord

Slow me down, Lord. Ease the pounding of my
    heart by the quieting of my mind.
Steady my hurried pace with a vision of the
    eternal reach of time.
Give me, amid the confusion of the day the
    calmness of the everlasting hills.
Break the tensions of my nerves and muscles
    with the soothing music of the singing
    streams that live in my memory.
Help me to know the magical, restoring power
    of sleep.
Teach me the art of taking minute vacations -
    of slowing down to look at a flower,
To chat with a friend, to pat a dog, to read a
    few lines from a good book.
Slow me down, Lord, and inspire me to send
    my roots deep into the soil of life's
    enduring values
That I may grow towards the stars of my
    greatest destiny.

Author Unknown

My Dad had always told me that I put such energy, more than the usual amount, into raising children. During those early years when the children were all under fourteen, I was a full time mother and wife and a part time health educator. I was always on the go!

What was this injury now trying to tell me? Was it that I probably needed some time off? In four days I was expected to drive to New York for Fleet Week to meet with our son aboard the USS America. Our soon to be daughter-in-law had been planning this for months. In fact five months earlier she chose to fly there, rather than take the chance that I might break my leg and not be able to drive! I won't even try to explain that one, except to say, that I was again so sad, knowing it was all out of my control.

The two of them called me from New York telling me that my room was ready and that they knew somehow that I would be there. I told them I could not spend eight hundred dollars on a last minute airplane ticket. My cast was up to my hip and it would not fit under the dash board of my mini van so I could not drive.

Overwhelmed, sitting back on the couch with my head so full of "stuff", I relaxed for a moment with a deep breath. This was just long enough for me to remember that my mail, which I had not read in the past two days, contained a letter from Northwest Airlines.

It was a frequent flyer ticket that had come in the day before. I was out of there! I knew that the world cared for the handicapped and besides New York City was going to be full of seven thousand sailors and my son, as my personal escort!

The airline was wonderful. My Husband was wonderful. The bus driver who got me to the hotel in New York was wonderful – all healers, helpers, wizards and guides.

I learned the magnificent power of a wheel chair. My Mom had walked on a walker for eight years. My Dad with one leg two inches shorter than the other walked with a cane for twenty-two years. I really did not feel I had to become like them to understand them, but there I was in full garb, with every ounce of their strength and determination inside of me.

I went by myself on my new crutches on this great adventure which lead me to climb on the deck of the U.S.S. America and down into the engine room where our son worked. Did we ever laugh a lot!

When my leg was almost healed, the orthopedic surgeon split my cast so that I could take it off and go swimming. It was summer. I only asked and promised not to walk on it without proper support. He and his staff were very special healers who touched my life at a vulnerable moment in a unique way.

When I returned home, I received a phone call from my gynecologist asking me to review my mammogram with a surgeon. They had found a spot on my left breast that needed to be removed.

In some ways I faced my own mortality when my parents passed away. This was real. I laughed when I broke my leg, but this was very serious. Too many of my friends had developed breast cancer and had died. What was to be my fate? Was I going to have to go through chemotherapy?

Refusing to total the stress points, I stayed in the present moment. I was past dealing with my life one day at a time. I was now handling about one minute at a time. My sisters were all sending me those wonderful cards that say, "We know you can make it. We love you!"

The surgeon removed the cyst which turned out to be benign, but the mind has a way of playing tricks on us. I had again let go of what I could not control and had accepted whatever was to befall me, only to not to have it happen. I was cleared, but even with all my positive beliefs, for the next few weeks after I still felt the anguish of those who had feared and had experienced the physical effects of chemotherapy.

> **The doctor, an osteopath recommended by my medical doctor, was wonderful beyond any expectation - spiritual, kind, loving and respectable.**

He was an incredible human being, who had turned fifty, lost his dear mother-in-law and broke his leg six months before! He knew my path well. Ironic is probably a good word, but there I was in his care with total unconditional love and support.

> **Healers, helpers, wizards and guides: such special people that come into our lives to help us through the most anguishing moments.**

The wedding was the high point of our summer. Shortly after, our son was shipped overseas and our youngest two children headed off to college. Our nest was truly empty for the first time in thirty years!

We had real mixed feelings, as we hoped that our life would settle down for a while. I was very tired and still had to have the steel plate removed from my ankle. Fortunately this was done without difficulty.

> **I was determined to take the time to heal whatever needed healing in me, the loss of both my parents, the broken leg, the breast surgery, the broken spirit, the empty nest. Whatever it was and whatever it took, I was going to do it.**

This had been a very full year to say the least. I wanted so much to get back to doing my workshops and seminars. My phone continued to ring. I had a great story to tell, and *Facing the Challenges of Change* turned out to be an honest title!

My new method of marketing took on the appearance of prayer. It was the best I could do that summer, but oh, the richness in spirit it brought to me! *Be Careful What You Pray For*, Larry Dossey says in his book of the same title. I began each day with the following reflection.

> **Dear God, send to me whoever needs what I have to share, or whoever has what You know I need. Help me to be open to receive whatever it is that will help me grow and heal. I will also trust that I will know when to speak and when to remain silent, as I reach out to others.**

CHAPTER THREE

It Was Only A Neck Injury, But Oh, How It Changed My Life!

Two winters ago I had acquired a form of asthma that was aggravated by exercise. I found that for the first time in my life, even if I only climbed stairs, I would cough. It was not like me to have this happen. I tried everything to get around it. Then I started on various inhalers. The four different types I tried terrified me in that I might need them for the rest of my life. None of them seemed to work.

Unfortunately, the doctor was unable to give me the information I felt I needed. "You'll have to live with it!" was an unacceptable answer to me. I wanted to find out the cause, and not just cover up the symptoms with medication. I went to another doctor, whose son had asthma as a child. He was very helpful. He was caring and very understanding and explained the physiology to me.

At least now I understood my choices and I had the chance to ask the right questions. I could exercise, but I had to take the medication before I began. I was also beginning to gain weight from lack of exercise, which became another concern to me.

I tried to stay positive and accepted my plight and locked into my computer to write the student-guide for my book, *Does Anyone Hear Our Cries for Help?*. Getting a good start on this before Christmas I trusted that my two weeks in Florida would cure whatever was happening in my lungs.

It was a great vacation - swimming, snorkeling walking, diving - all with my husband. Kids were content with their jobs and with the families of their boyfriends and girlfriends. We had celebrated Christmas at Thanksgiving and we were feeling very grateful for these two weeks alone taking care of ourselves! What more could I want?

After our holiday, we returned to Michigan to the grey skies and cold weather. I love Michigan and I don't mind winter here, especially, when I dress warm. But the asthma came back and so did some seasonal depression!

I would tell myself, "I'm in charge of me and I am not going to let this get me down." I wasn't winning. I was feeling older, and more tired.

At times I felt as if I were sleeping to catch up on all the sleep I had lost in my lifetime. I could not believe how much this body needed its sleep.

I was falling into a pattern I didn't like. I wanted to do something different. I enjoyed writing the activity guidebook, but I love being outdoors and the sun was shining, so I went ice skating. I had skated most of my life, as a child, on a pond near our home on Long Island. That's what we all did in the winter, as teenagers. It was the place to gather with friends.

Feeling awkward, at first, I practiced skating at a park nearby where no one could see me, except for a few kids who didn't care. After a half hour, I was right back skating where I had left off fifteen years ago.

I only fell a few times that day. These falls seemed to be uneventful except that I remember saying, as I slid sprawled eagle across the ice, "Oh! Maybe these days I should be wearing a helmet, as I do when I use my bike." But this was just a thought.

Later, I realized that I had a whiplash injury to my neck that day. This caused in me that notorious stiff neck that so many of us live with as a silent injury. I chose to ignore the discomfort for many months, believing that it would go away. My denial came from my strong belief that in time this would heal on its own.

> **I gave the injury time to get better. Six months later it had not healed and the movement in my neck had become greatly limited.**

I did not want to ask for anymore help. "Aren't I strong enough yet?" I would ask myself. "Was this just another sign of weakness?" I was sure it was time for me to be all better. Did I have to give into the belief that I might need support from other people again?

I really wanted to get on with my life. I was being hard on myself, but I was feeling so immobilized. My passion to facilitate my seminars and workshops was still there, but I couldn't get the fires going to make it work again as a business.

> **I again began to think that maybe this was all part of the aging process. Wasn't this why people retire?**

I was also going through peri-menopause with all the symptoms that go with it. Dr. Christiane Northrup, M.D., in her wonderful book, *Woman's Bodies, Woman's Wisdom,* says that "this time (peri-menopause) represents the early years of change in a woman's menstrual cycle before menopause. During this time a woman gradually stops ovulating and her ovaries slow down the production of estrogen and progesterone." This is actually a very special time for women to return to self and evaluate where they have been so far in life and where they will go in the second half of their lives.

These feelings and the experiences of physical weakness, fluid retention, fatigue, hot flashes and decreased mental clarity were all very real to me. I also knew that this was a big part of my picture. I had already made the decision not to take hormone replacement. My older sisters had told me that these symptoms would only last a few years.

I couldn't think in those numbers. I could only handle a day here and a day there. Heart palpitations, dry skin, short term forgetfulness, tiredness and hot flashes - would they ever go away?

> **My mom had an eight and ten year old child (me) and three teenagers when she was my age. How did she ever do it? Where had my energy gone? I wanted it back.**

Finally, spring came and we got our boats in the water. I found myself out racing on our small sailboat with my husband. All of sudden the mainsail boom jibed and hit me on the side of the head doing a major adjustment to the cervical vertebrae of my neck. I did not break anything, but things were not too good. Now, I really had a stiff neck!

Oh well! Such is life! It was now time to have this neck injury checked out. Besides, the stiffness from the winter skating outing had really never gone away.

> **It's interesting how long it takes, sometimes, for us to face the realities of our health. As Paul Pearsall says in his book, *Super Immunity*, "Illness is not in your head, but almost all wellness is."**

Fear of the unknown and actually not wanting to know the truth, kept me from taking the time to check out my neck sooner. At this point the only choice I had left was to take care of the problem with outside help or suffer the consequences forever.

**This decision to take care of me was the begin-
ning of one of the most incredible healing journeys I have ever undertaken.**

Our son and my husband had received great results in
Chiropractic care. I too believed in their basic philosophy of
going after the cause of an injury and allowing the natural
forces within the body to heal itself. I had experienced both
the medical perspective and the chiropractic approach to this
type of injury about ten years ago.

At that time, I had excellent success with a different
Chiropractor after being unhappy for six months on medications that only covered up the pain and made me sleepy. I
was therefore comfortable, at this point, with taking on the
challenge to find an alternative path to being cured.

**Whenever I asked anyone how they felt about
their experiences in Chiropractic care, they always
answered with such positive love and sense of
connection.**

Recently, I heard an interesting statistic indicating that a
very large number of patients today are combining alternative means of healing therapies with their medical care, but
not bothering to tell their medical doctors. I was certain that
the reason for this was their belief that there should be a
happy marriage between the two and, as a patient, they did
not want to be the arbitrator in the controversy.

On my first visit to the Chiropractor, I found out more
than I wanted to know. There were many empty places in my
life that I was trying to fill up. A lot had happened to me all
at once.

**I was addicted to chocolate. I had become careless
with my health and I was eating the wrong foods.
If I was not careful, I could be eating all the time.**

I believed I was strong spiritually and that I was doing everything I could do to bring my strength and energy back. After all, I'm a motivational speaker and health educator. Shouldn't I be listening to my own tapes and reading my own books?

I also knew there were a lot of things that I wasn't doing. A regular program of exercise was one of them because of the asthma. I was also eating to fill up the emptiness caused by the changes and losses in my life. These were major issues. I had moved into a form of passive resignation believing that things had to be as they were. I had given most of my energy away and I was tired – always tired, but not in public!

In many ways I had allowed the world out there to influence my thoughts of whom I was to become, as I grew older.

The following statistics need to be shared with everyone, men and women alike.

Did you know…?

- There are three billion women who don't look like super models and only eight who do.
- Marilyn Monroe wore a size twelve dress.
- The average American woman weighs one hundred and forty-four pounds and wears between a size twelve and fourteen.
- One out of every four college-aged women has an eating disorder.
- If shop mannequins were real women they'd be too thin to menstruate.
- The models in the magazines are airbrushed— They are not perfect!!
- If Barbie were a real woman, she'd have to walk on all fours due to her proportions.

- A psychological study in 1995 found that three minutes spent looking at models in a fashion magazine caused seventy percent of women to feel depressed, guilty and shameful.
- Models who, twenty years ago, weighed eight percent less than the average woman, today weigh twenty-three percent less.

There is no reason why our generation of women and future generations should destroy their bodies and their health to look thin. They are simply being lied to. We can all learn to love ourselves for who we are and not for what others think we should look like.

I began to focus on the health of my whole body and not just on my weight.

This was probably the one main reason I chose to write this book. We are a world full of excuses for not taking care of ourselves. My list runs long. I've known all the rules. I've taught them for years. I had moved them onto the back burner out of sight for a while. But now, it was time to bring them back to the forefront. I had to say to myself, "I'm done with all my excuses. I alone will accept the consequences of my choices." If I want to feel better, I am the only one who can make it happen. This time I meant it.

I missed the people who had given me so much unconditional love, even though there were others to help fill that emptiness. It wasn't the same. Some empty spaces could not be filled. They just needed to heal.

Unconditional love is such an awesome gift - love that has no conditions - love that accepts others "exactly as they are in all their magnificence", as Arnold Patent clearly expresses in his book, *You Can Have It All*.

The doctor's assessment and evaluation was completed. I didn't really know the Doctor. He was a Doctor of Chiropractic who uses the Activator Method of treatment to facilitate healing through proper alignment of my spine and my neck vertebrae. He was a specialist in subluxation, or misaligned vertebrae, who, as the Chiropractic literature says, "works with the body and its Creator to accelerate the healing process that naturally takes place within each of us."

I wasn't quite sure what that all meant, but I knew that this healing process also had something to do with bringing all the components of the mind, body, and spirit into balance. I did know that he had been putting our athletic son back together for two years and that our son thought he was awesome!

My husband also had confidence in him and was definitely feeling better following his car accident a year ago. His blood pressure also had returned to normal. They were both good indicators that I was in the right place.

On the X-ray the doctor found that apparently, many years ago, I had a whiplash injury to my neck. As a result, I had a reversed "S" curve in my neck. All these years I never knew the injury was there. The stiffness had been activated by my skating and sailing accidents. That was the bad news. He said that it was pretty serious. The good news was that he could fix it.

That was it! If this doctor could do what he said he could do, then I would work with him and do what I had to do to make my injured neck better. One adjustment at a time each visit, I began to put my life back together.

At this point I had no idea how this injury had affected my life through the years, but I was about to find out. With blind faith based on the assurance of two reputable family members, I found myself in the chiropractor's office three days a week.

> **Straight out the doctor had told me with total certitude and twenty-five years experience, "I can fix it!" Why would he say he could, if he couldn't?**

Was this a chance for me to be my humble self, who would allow me to accept the care I truly needed from another human being?

> **Was this person to give me back the balance in my life that I had somehow misplaced along the way? The answer to this was, "Yes, it was time for a vacation - a vacation inward in silence." I needed it all: mind, body, spirit.**

It was important to me to make the choice to stay committed to my Chiropractic program, whatever that was. The initial intensive care had something to do with taking away the physical pain, my headaches and the stiffness in my neck and shoulders. At the time it seemed like this pain was everywhere throughout my body. I was totally aware of its presence and my limitation in physical movement. I knew this process of healing meant more than just taking this away. This would also involve rehabilitative care to stabilize the spine and repair muscle and soft tissue damage.

I began this journey taking full responsibility for its outcome. No one but me, could be the voice of my injury. It was my choice to care for my health and I knew it.

> **This became a journey backwards in time that has lead me to places I never thought I would revisit with the same vitality of those days long gone. In other words, I feel younger and so much lighter, even though my weight has not changed...yet!**

CHAPTER FOUR

Getting Centered

I never stopped asking questions. I made up my mind, that if I were going to drive thirty-five minutes each way, three days a week, then I was going to make it count. I wasn't sure what I was counting. I was really feeling in a bad way when this part of my healing journey began. The following list describes my feelings at that time:

disconnected	uncomfortable	alone
depressed	old and aging	heavy
empty	immobilized	hungry
annoyed	controlled	injured
out of balance	insecure	in pain
fearful	vulnerable	weak
distracted	hungry	humble
tired	preoccupied	forgetful

Six months later those feelings had been transformed into the following:

strong	balanced	happy
empowered	peaceful	prayerful
loving	content	positive
spiritual	rested	caring
empathetic	centered	excited
motivated	satisfied	energized
limitless	enthusiastic	free spirited
attentive	calm	joyful

Now the question is: how did I get there in six months? To begin with, I realized the importance of getting centered on why I was in the care of this doctor.

In high school I had a Biology teacher who was one of my special guides throughout much of my formal education. Everyone loved Ernie and everyone wanted to be in his classes.

I asked him a few years ago, if he ever knew how unique he was in those days. He said, "I was told that for many years by my colleagues and students. The only thing that I could attribute this to was that each day as I went off to work, I centered myself on my purpose and mission in life and carried that awareness into my classroom and into my relationships."

As his student, I may not remember the specific science lessons he taught me, but I can tell you that his classroom was always safe for me to be myself. This powerful experience taught me what was possible for all of us when we set proper boundaries and allow this to happen. We all want to find that place of safety in our lives where we can be ourselves.

With each visit to the chiropractor's office as soon as I arrived, no matter what mental acrobatics I had to perform, I would do the following:

- Sit quietly, relax and connect with the healing process
- Let go of any issue of time
- Focus on a point of center within my body
- Clear my head of its daily clutter
- Focus on my purpose for being there in the care of this doctor
- Pray for the guidance of the doctor's hands
- Let go of all my questions of the week
- Trust that whatever I needed to know would be answered after the adjustment
- Let go of any expectation that anything should be other than it is

- Remain quiet within and listen for the sounds of learning
- Feel the safety of the moment to be myself
- Let go of the outcome and watch the healing process unfold (This last one took a while for me to understand.)

Becoming centered had a pleasant effect on my whole being. It gave me some quiet time to reflect before the doctor came in. Each visit I cleared my head of my questions and quietly prayed to know which one was most important in my healing journey for that day. It was always the right question because I accepted whatever came and the answer that followed would take me to the next level of understanding. It was good to practice and affected other areas of my life, as well.

Without the mental clutter created by unfulfilled expectations, each visit then became as perfect as it was meant to be. What a lesson it was for me each time to let go of the outcome. It took a while. I also believed that whatever it was that the doctor needed to hear from me was also said. I had many visits to practice this over the next few months. Without worrying about what I wanted to say, I could truly remain focused on my healing.

When we begin each day by getting centered, focusing on the present moment and our purpose for being, it helps us to pay attention and to keep out the negativity and other distractions. Worry only takes energy away from the healing process.

As we go through the day defending ourselves, we don't always realize how certain self-defeating attitudes affect our behavior. They can wear us down and rob us of our positive energy. Learning to detach by focusing and getting centered is a choice we can make that will make a difference to us.

I had used this same technique to prepare myself and become centered before I began teaching or facilitating a workshop, seminar, or presenting a keynote address. I knew that the doctor, even with his wonderful sense of humor, took the adjustment time very seriously. He had even asked that, as his patients, we remain silent and present to our healing, as he worked. I also prayed for the guidance of his hands and connected with that process.

To bring myself back to center throughout the day, I often remind myself of the following:

1. I will stay in the present moment and not become overwhelmed with all of life's problems.

2. I will remember to keep positive healing thoughts in my head and move any self-defeating ones away.

3. I will keep my mind, heart and ears open and accept others as they are without judgment.

4. I will accept myself as I am and do my best at whatever I do.

5. I will take time for the small things in life slowing down to acknowledge and accept my good feelings.

6. I will greet others with the same kindness and love that I wish for myself.

7. I will let go of my expectations for other people to be other than who they are and accept their choices.

8. I will let go of the anxiety and stress attached to time and accept that where I am now is where I belong. I will trust God's time in the healing process.

9. And finally, I will take time to listen to my own inner voice and ask for guidance through my life journey.

Sometimes in my silence, I would also remind myself that the world out there may never understand the way I do things. What was important was that I understood and accepted myself as I am. I did not allow myself to compare myself to anyone else. If I did, it would only slow me down and inhibit me from finding the clarity and peace of mind I was so desperately looking for.

I came to understand the answer to, "Do you really like the company you keep in quiet moments?" I was beginning to recognize my need for solitude in order to get my strength back. These feelings were hitting me from all directions. In the safety of the adjustment room of the doctor's office, I began blocking out the disconnected noises "out there" in the world. From there I expanded this experience to include other places in my life.

What is this injury asking me to do? What did I fear and why? What life-giving change was about to happen to me? Becoming centered was going to give my body a chance to answer those questions, if I would listen.

I thought I understood the silent part of this journey, but in the farthest stretch of my imagination, I could never have realized its power.

I was ready to listen!

CHAPTER FIVE

One Person's Journey
Through Chiropractic Care

When I began Chiropractic care, I had just completed my annual physical with my medical doctors. My blood work, blood pressure, pap smear and mammogram were all excellent, but I knew that deep within this body of mine something was not right. What had this crooked neck created in me for so long?

I had been living on an emotional roller coaster for over three years, unable to focus or function clearly with any direction. Beyond the symptoms of peri-menopause, I always felt like I was climbing uphill with a physical resistance connected to most of my movements. I felt as if I was viewing life through opaque lenses. Some days my headaches completely took over my day along with the pain in my shoulders and neck.

I pretended not to let it bother me. I did not feel balanced or strong anymore. I was unhappy about that. I reminded myself daily that I was finally taking care of it. I tried not to concentrate on the pain and focused instead on the good things that were happening.

The very first change I noticed in the first week of Chiropractic care was that I got my sense of smell back. It had been gone for many years. Actually, that's not such a bad thing when you have three kids in diapers! But those days are long gone and now it would be good to know if something was burning on the stove!

Only twenty percent returned at first. The rest of my sense of smell came back completely about eight months later, after more than twenty years. I was like a kid in a candy store walking through my mother-in-law's beautiful flower garden the week it happened. The aroma from the lilacs, the roses, the peppermint and spearmint was wonderful. It was like the return of an old friend long gone.

Ironically, the second thing that came back, I wasn't looking for, and that was my menstrual cycle. The Chiropractor said that often happens to many women in Chiropractic care. It had something to do with the fact that, as the vertebrae of the spine become properly aligned, the flow of fluids through the body is no longer inhibited. I had been retaining water for months. This bloating was very obvious in a driver's license photo that was taken that month and again retaken four months later after I had misplaced it.

Whatever was not working right then, was again working now, as it should. I felt good about that.

When my menstrual cycle ended this time, it stopped properly and with much more peacefulness, leaving only power surges of heat, as hot flashes, to replace it. These did not bother me at all. I was intrigued. I was definitely beginning to feel better from my weekly visits. For the hot flashes that sometimes seemed endless, I created a wonderful visual.

I looked at them, as energy fields of love surrounding me. It was time now for me to love myself and to take care of me. This gave me a chance to feel the embrace. It worked well for me, like a quiet meditation, as I continued on this journey.

The muscles of my neck and upper back continued to hurt. I understood that, as these were strengthened to pull the vertebrae from another direction, they would become tender from having not been used for a while. This soreness was what I was feeling. Neglected injuries often cause the body to adjust improperly, shifting it out of balance. As these body parts were being reprogrammed, there occurred a time when everything inside me seemed to be in a state of confusion.

This compared to the way I felt the first few days each spring, when I began conditioning for running, a sport I had not done for five years. I had not exercised much for over a year and maybe even longer because of the asthma.

As the weeks went by, I felt like I was always in training. I never realized how long it would take to rebuild the muscles in my neck. I kept at it, trusting and working hard to be patient, but I wanted it done yesterday!

I was doing the assigned isometrics to strengthen my neck muscles. My head was actually beginning to feel as if it were no longer connected to my shoulders for whatever reason. It was very strange, for there was no discomfort. This lasted about two weeks and then finally stabilized in the fourth week. The mobility of my neck had not changed. The stiffness was there and my side movement was still very limited.

I had no idea where this was going to lead me. I was on a quest. It had become important to me to take care of my health and to get back on track. I chose not to be frightened by the physical process, whatever that was, and trusted the "facilitator of my healing," my doctor. I could feel his confidence.

I stayed with it. I kept trusting my instincts, my gut feelings, that told me that I was seeing, what I was feeling.

It is a strange way to explain it, but I had to be a "patient patient" yet speak my concerns, which I never stopped doing, even when I found myself taking the risk to push myself through my fears. I began to have many questions.

Where were all these questions coming from? I was a health educator for years. Was it all so new to me, or was it so familiar that I wanted to know more? Was I "asleep" during all those years? I don't think so.

Sometimes I would wonder what other patients thought, but I learned long ago that I could only pay attention to my own needs and that was a big enough job in itself. To say I was preoccupied with all that was happening around me and inside of me would be an understatement. I was beginning to wear down.

That which is not addressed in life begs attention. New emotions of sadness were coming out of nowhere. I was very tired of the physical resistance I was feeling. I did not want to quit. I just wanted the pain to go away.

Somehow, throughout my life there have been many incongruities of love and hate among those closest to me. I could never control the behaviors of others, yet, somehow I thought I should have been able to. No matter how I tried to rescue them from their pain, I somehow always seemed to end up in the middle. I never could pacify or understand it. I usually ended up owning the problem as if it were somehow my fault.

I spent visit after visit letting go of what I could not control in my life and trying to silence the noises in my head that were asking all the questions. I knew my physical pain was connected to my emotional pain.

Then the following dream happened to me. It was so real that I accepted the peace it brought to me. I remembered the words I heard that morning many times during the ensuing months.

My Dream

It was early in the morning. The alarm had just gone off and my husband had gotten up. I did not wake up but instead found myself standing outside of the cellar door of the home I grew up in on Long Island. I could hear my dad through the basement door calling me. I went inside. He was sitting on the cellar steps about the third step up.

He called to me saying, "Come here, Baby."

I walked over to him and I brushed back his pure white hair on this bald head and gently touched the sides of his face saying, "You look so beautiful, Daddy, and so at peace."

"Come here, Baby." He said again, gently, as he reached out to put his arms around me and held me, as he did so many times in my life and said, "Don't you worry, Baby, everything is going to be all right."

I felt so at peace with him, as he comforted me. I felt all of his loving energy. I knew he was there, and if he wasn't, it didn't matter because I got the message. With renewed faith I was determined to go through the pain because I knew that it was what I was supposed to do.

My dad's reassurance told me that I could continue to trust. I was doing something he so much wanted to do himself, when he was alive. He had been my cheerleader. He often shared his stories of letting go. One time was when my mom was sick with encephalitis when I was very young. Then again two years later, he had to let go when he broke his hip in a major car accident. He had been my pillar of strength in my life and I knew I was to keep on going.

> It takes such courage to trust that you will make it through all that is being asked of you at any moment in your life. This "letting go" is what creates the spiritual awakening. It was all part of this healing process of reconnecting the mind, body and spirit. I knew I would have to continue to trust.

What an extreme responsibility one gives to others in whom you instill your trust, as your healer, helper, wizard or guide. Where is their integrity of intention? Who is their God? What if money is their God? Be it a president, a therapist, a teacher, a medical doctor, osteopath, chiropractor, practitioner, mother, father, or friend - what an incredible responsibility to work within the boundaries of integrity and trust! What if they forget who they are?

If these individuals have the power to heal, they also have the power to injure and, if fame and fortune are their god, and they choose to injure for their own satisfaction or for the sake of more money, how sad for them and how sad for all of us, who place our trust in them! For those who are given many gifts, much is expected.

> Also then, what about touch? My friend and mentor, Sidney Simon, author of the book, *Caring, Feeling, Touching,* says that "The secret of touch is in the intentionality. We must always remember that the person we touch is someone's baby and he or she must be touched with reverence. The intentionality comes from knowing that these hands are my sexual hands and they are also my healing hands that put band-aids on wounded

children. They are also the hands that have comforted a dying mother and the hands that have massaged the tiredness from the body of my love partner. Intentionality is the secret."

If I give people the honor of my trust, my expectation is that they will uphold that trust with impeccable integrity. I know that this can only exist in an ideal world. I also believe that a global healing, bringing us world peace and harmony, cannot take place until we all heal ourselves first. We must remain committed to communicate in a way that helps us to let go of the judgments that drive us apart. With this commitment in our collective consciousness we can bring about world peace.

To create a relationship of trust we can:
- listen with our heart
- share our "personal story" that brought us to our calling
- be human and show our sensitive side
- engage in kindness and compassion
- be consistent with clear boundaries
- model impeccable integrity of intention
- pay attention to body language
- make eye contact without fear of what others may be thinking
- trust ourselves to know what we know

When I was younger I truly believed that I could only trust certain people until I caught them in a lie. Now that I have raised my family and have experienced half a lifetime full of many healers, helpers, wizards and guides, I now know that I can trust those I choose to trust. If, or when I catch them in a lie, I will forgive them and then let it go. On one such occasion when I felt sadness from a misunderstanding with a friend, I wrote the following:

He Hurt Me!

He hurt me!
He didn't know he did it,
but he did.
He hurt me when I felt
I didn't deserve it.

I wanted to tell him how
and why it hurt so much.
I wanted to tell him
it wasn't the first time.

I wanted to tell him all
in every detail, but I didn't.
I somehow felt he knew.
I somehow trusted that we've been
close friends a long time.

I somehow knew he was sorry.
So I just forgave him.

© 1998 Bertie Synowiec

The poem reflects the way I handle things now with non-judgment. It is part of what I was learning in silence at the time. In the poem I chose to feel hurt. I could also choose not to feel hurt and not to take it personally. Maybe in my heart I was feeling the hurtful stories of others and wrote it as a form of hope for me - that everything need not be explained. Some things just are what they are. True healing involves forgiveness.

I showed the poem to my husband in terms of our relationship. Now we talk out our personal issues with love and forgiveness rather than defensiveness. The wisdom is in the ability to move beyond the words into the heart of what is not being said. The "he" represents those people in our lives, who hurt us automatically with no intention connected to the behavior.

As John Bradshaw, author of *Bradshaw: On The Family: A Revolutionary Way of Self-Discovery*, says, "Guilt gives us a conscience. When I say something to hurt you, I have a feeling about that. I've done something to hurt you. When I lose that conscience, then I don't see other people's discomfort as real. When we embrace the feelings, it brings us to our reality. Without feelings we have no reality. Sharing our feelings brings us closer to one another."

I like to believe that. It makes it easier to forgive those who may not be connected to their feelings.

One by one I faced my fears directly. For me headaches, chronic pain and emotional crisis all came with the healing package, as the nerve pressure was being released. I knew I was where I belonged. I began to make myself accountable to myself and what health goals I wanted to set for myself. This released my determination.

Getting physically stronger became my primary focus. I began to swim. I continued to walk. I was easy on me. I had many things to do to get well. I stayed in the present moment.

I did not want to get frustrated, nor did I want to feel that I had to do anything unless it was comfortable for me. I walked if I felt like it, or biked. Whatever I was in the mood to do, I did. Summertime would make it easier. Or does it? I now know that is only an excuse. Forty degree weather is not too cold when I am dressed warmly and walking quickly.

Trying not to do all things at once, I instead chose one goal each week to work on. Time became irrelevant.

Dr. Andrew Weil's book, *Eight Weeks to Optimum Health* entered my life. He said "to breathe!" Oh my goodness what a novel idea! "Eat greens. Eat healthy. Walk ten minutes. Go on a news fast and then decide how much news you really want in your life."

I was way ahead of him on that one. I had made the decision back in the 60's to limit my intake of that sensationalism, after the assassinations of all those wonderful guides who were our governmental leaders. I do not do well with that kind of news, so why feed on it.

Dr. Weil's suggestions were easy for me to fit into a week, when I still was not be sure about how much I wanted to do. I was on a roll!

I also read and listened to many relevant books. One in particular, *The Celestine Prophecy* by James Redford gave me great reassurance. So many unexplainable things were happening to me. I think I was looking for new insights!

I was beginning to get of my energy back. It was still early. I was eating more salads and fruit. I would make them ahead of time and have them available in my refrigerator, so as to help me avoid other foods that were not as healthy.

My husband and I both decided to supplement our food intake with a vitamin/mineral tonic. There are many to choose from on the market. We both believed that taking this made a big difference, even if only to build our security around the issue of getting all the right vitamins and minerals into our foods.

With this supplement I also found that I began to lose my cravings, something I was very glad to have out of my life. It was strange, but I no longer felt like I had to eat all the time. I continued to focus on the health of my whole body.

I also began to drink water. It sounds strange to put it that way, but like my mother before me, I basically drank coffee. Only my coffee was decaffeinated. I somehow thought water was boring and I never cared for pop, or soda. Besides, I never could figure out how I could get eight glasses of water into me and still be able to find a bathroom!

Well, I figured it out from a health guide I received from the doctor's office, only I did it my way because it worked better for me. I drank one glass in the morning, when I first got up. Then I would have my decaffeinated coffee. As time went on, I dropped the coffee and switched to a diluted decaffeinated tea with some honey in it. Since my energy was definitely coming back through Chiropractic care, I did not need the pick up from the coffee. Also tea never got bitter, even if it sat for a while.

At noon I would drink half of a thirty-two ounce water bottle, filtered from the faucet to remove chemical impurities. Remember, life is about choices. Distilled water was even more boring to me and I really knew drinking water was good for me so I compromised! I would then have my lunch. Shortly after, I would drink the other half of the bottle, another sixteen ounces. The second twenty-four ounce bottle, I would put in my car for later that afternoon when I was on my way home. This way I was able to drink my eight (eight ounce) glasses of water each day.

Before I started doing this I was always thirsty because of my busy schedule. By late evening I would drink enough to make me have to get up in the middle of the night. This new way worked well for me and my skin was no longer dry. It also had a certain glow to it, that it had not seen in many years!

The combination of the mineral and vitamin tonic, sixty-four ounces of water, exercise and the Chiropractic visits on a regular schedule were making a big difference in my life.

With my injury I was given the gift of time - the time to heal - even though time was such an issue for those still creating schedules. I began to look at time only as something other people scheduled!

I relaxed more. I was now facing many challenges of change in my life and wrote the following to help me along my path.

Facing the Challenges of Change

1. I will take the risk to change and trust that I am not alone. No one is asking me to compromise my values.

2. Change stretches me beyond my comfort zone and gives me an opportunity to learn and experience new things.

3. Change begins with me. I cannot change another person. I can only change myself. Love them anyway!

4. I will let go of what I cannot control. As long as I hold on to the old ways of doing things, there will be no room for what is new.

5. I must stay in the present moment and recognize that right where I am is where I am supposed to be!

6. When I begin to feel overwhelmed, I will take a break. I will stop and reflect to clear my head and begin again.

7. All I get done in one day is all that I am supposed to do!

8. Who I am does not depend on what other people may think of me. They need not understand. I can take care of myself and adapt to change my own way.

9. I have every right to ask questions, even when someone does not understand that right.

10. I will trust my instincts and my ability to learn new techniques. The outcome is what is important, as I begin to understand the new procedures.

11. I can be patient with me! Slow isn't bad. Fast isn't better and different isn't wrong™. We all have our own special way of learning things. Fear of being "graded" or "judged" only slows us down.

12. I will turn change into an ally so that I can embrace it rather than resist it.

13. If I do not like something or someone, I can change my attitude towards that person or situation.

14. Gently I will accept the challenges of change and know that I have the ability to manage them one step at a time. Fighting them will only exhaust me.

CHAPTER SIX

Personal Challenges To Change: Symptom Or Cause

According to the Encyclopedia of Alternative Medicines, edited by Jennifer Jacobs, M.D. MPH, 1997 and endorsed by the American Holistic Health Association, "Chiropractic is now the world's largest drug-free healing profession with over 50,000 practitioners, licensed in all 50 states, as Doctors of Chiropractic. They are considered primary health care providers.

Attempts to compare Chiropractic to traditional medicine creates an "apples and oranges" situation. Each is different. Each has its own strengths and place.

- **Medical care is effective in crisis care, emergency treatment for trauma, accident, disease and immediate life threatening conditions.**

- **Chiropractic enhances the health of the individual by correcting nerve interference (vertebral subluxation). Chiropractors do not attempt to treat disease, although many specific conditions heal with Chiropractic care."**

Remaining healthy is a life process according to Chiropractic. It's philosophy is health based, rather than disease based. Paying attention and doing healthy things on a regular basis allows the patient to create a lifestyle that focuses on the signs of good health while the chiropractor works with our body's natural innate intelligence to keep us healthy at all times.

Traditional medicine correctly teaches us to observe the signs of a disease, such as in looking for signs of cancer. For optimal health and wellness there needs to be a combination of both the traditional disease forces of medicine and the modern open-ended health focus of Chiropractic.

Without this simple understanding among health professionals, doctors may choose to believe that they are in competition for the same patients. I have a great concern when I see this. I have watched this for years within our educational system, as school counselors and outside counseling agencies competed for the same funding for certain services provided to children. Instead of a collaborative effort, these resources have not always been available to the child who needs the services.

This happens within the medical profession when certain individuals with wonderful gifts criticize the wisdom and philosophy of Chiropractic care. I have always been uncomfortable with this discordance. There is no reason for this. It is a disservice to the patients who are seeking the best care for themselves, or their family.

Each has its place. But for overall health, it makes so much more sense for health care professionals to look for the underlying cause of an illness or injury. The answer may not be to medicate the symptoms with drugs.

I am a scientist. I understand the necessity for research based data. But the proof is there and it is time to stop pretending it is not. Studies have shown that continued Chiropractic care for certain injuries provides better outcomes in the healing process than can be provided by the medical profession. With managed health care deciding the amount of time a doctor can spend with a patient, we are fast becoming our own teachers and choosing our own paths to good health. This is expressed in the following statistic:

One third of all Americas (66 million) using
orthodox medicine are also using some form of
alternative therapy and pay 10.4 billion dollars
out of pocket to access alternative therapy that
they cannot get elsewhere. Sometimes this is only
to access relationship." David Eisenburg. *New
England Journal of Medicine. Survey On The Use
Of Alternative Therapy Medical Interventions,*
1993.

Many medical doctors still base their views toward
alternative therapy on misinformation and throw all forms of
alternative medicine into the same pile. They just do not
realize that most of us would travel to the ends of the earth to
be with a doctor who understands the mindbodyspirit relationship and who is willing to connect with his or her patients at the heart.

When we are injured, frightened and hurting, we want
the security of someone who will listen to us as equals and
not as "weaklings" because we are ill or injured. We want a
doctor who doesn't have to think he, or she, is God and who
would not be afraid to take the time to teach us what we may
not understand.

**A good doctor with a supportive, caring practice
never has an empty parking lot!**

Why wouldn't we want to feel our best and have all the
parts of our body functioning in harmony? Why wouldn't we
want the mindbodyspirit connection working, as it was
created to be? With my neck injury I had already made the
decision not to go the route of medicating the symptoms. I
chose instead to enter Chiropractic care, to locate and correct
the cause of my discomfort.

There is another side to this in the same perspective. It is also unfair for doctors of chiropractic to expect a patient with many years of medical orientation to drop this conditioning the minute they walk in the door searching for this new holistic approach to the healing process.

Who is to be the teacher for this change? How can we, as patients, pull from within, information to which we may never have been exposed?

Why not ask a new patient the name of their family doctor and then ask permission to send the doctor a short report or update on their diagnosis and treatment along with a cover letter? Good communications helps create positive working relationships, as each party takes the risk to change without concern for what others may say, or think about them.

Attitudes and Approaches of Doctors

The old way:
- stay in control
- do not get involved
- stay detached emotionally
- shield themselves from the pain
- give limited responses controlled by time
- answer only questions asked
- set up the rules and conditions for care
- predict end results, if rules are not followed
- be fully responsible for healing/curing the illness
- create limitations for accessibility
- see no need in teaching the patient
- remain smarter than the patient
- maintain formal body language
- keep patients in their place

The new way:
- put patient needs first
- establish a partnership of equality
- believe healing is never predictable
- facilitate the natural process of healing
- empower patient's ownership of the process
- maintain trust within the healing relationship
- believe in the mindbodyspirit connection
- be the teacher for prevention
- be the model for good healthy choices
- explain the process or program
- be sensitive to feelings and concerns
- look directly into the eyes without fear
- listen with the heart to learn from them
- remove all resistance in body language
- understand need to grieve loss of function
- listen to understand fears
- offer compassion, hope and reassurance
- put patients in charge of their lives
- keep patient informed of progress

Bernie Siegel, M.D., in his book, *Love, Miracles and Medicine* **says, "We should be studying the exceptional patient, the successful patient instead of the failures. Exceptional patients:**

- **refuse to feel sorry for themselves.**
- **educate themselves and**
- **become a specialist in their own care.**
- **demand that their doctor take on the role of teacher.**
- **take responsibility for the outcome of their illness and health."**

Fifteen years ago in all my co-dependent craziness, I honestly did not know that my life could be anything but what it was. It was all I had ever known, even though it seemed so wrong. It was a medical doctor, a wonderfully spiritual, unconditionally loving human being and friend, who made it safe enough for me to take the risk to share my anguish. He was a true healer in every way. Without judgment he reached out to me and helped me begin a different journey towards inner peace.

While raising the children, I had been pulled into the belief that when the children were sick they always needed some form of medication to get better. In those days the availability of medicine greatly reduced my fears that something would happen to my children.

Whatever happened to my belief in the natural healing process of the body? At times these medications were important, but for us far more prescriptions than necessary were written. Not every doctor did this, nor did every parent get caught up in this but I know I did. We were told that they were dispensed, as preventive medicine, for possible bacterial infections that often occurred along with the viral infection.

What did I know? At the time I didn't know enough to ask the question and little or no information was given to me regarding side effects. Today prescriptions come with a very informative explanation. Also many of us can access the prescription desk reference.

My dad lived to be almost ninety when no one else in his family before him lived past sixty-two. Prescribed medicines helped reduce his high blood pressure. Chiropractic care would probably have helped his high blood pressure stabilize, as it helped my husband, but we did not know that then.

Medications are important in emergency situations. They should never be abused. I only needed to have a nephew at seven months old come down with spinal meningitis and then to have my own child, ten years old, fall thirty-

five feet from a willow tree onto his head, to know the importance of surgery and prescription drugs and the caring
dedication of the wonderful healers that prescribed them.

**I truly admire the doctor who chooses to integrate
the wisdom and philosophies of alternative
medicine and prescribed medicine into their
practices.**

There can be, and in time there will be, a marriage
between the two. In many circles it is already happening.
Some are even working out of the same offices. This collabo-
ration also occurs when the Chiropractor goes with his or her
patient to the surgeon or medical doctor when that is necessary. In my case it was my medical doctor, an obstetrician,
that recommended a very gifted osteopath to perform the
biopsy on my breast.

Attitudes of Patients:

The old way:
- believes the doctor is all-knowing
- is totally submissive to what they are told
- follows all the rules
- takes medicine
- does not ask questions
- trusts the doctor without question

The new way:
Patients want a doctor or practitioner who:
- understands the healing process
- will access relationship
- is emotionally supportive of feelings
- spends time with them
- shows compassion and understanding
- has high integrity

- gives information and reassurance
- encourages the patient to do their part
- lets patient be responsible for the outcome
- is accessible in times of fear or need
- is someone who believes in them
- provides resources for questions asked
- gives safe haven to be self
- is non-judgmental and accepting
- uses correct Biology in explaining problems
- gives clear directions
- gives positive encouragement for healthiness
- is a resource for tapes, books, booklets
- allows positive choices for best care

I have many doctor friends and I have been fascinated
by their response to my decision to stay in Chiropractic care.
Openness to change comes with letting go of our fears and
trusting a system that projects such caring sensitivity to the
needs of the patient. Those that have taken the time to do
this, through their own personal growth, were so open and
encouraging to me. This included my neurologist who had
done the surgery on our son twenty years ago.

> **Don't walk in front of me.**
> **I may not follow.**
> **Don't walk behind me.**
> **I may not lead.**
> **Walk beside me**
> **And just be my friend.**
> **Author Unknown**

Other health care professionals, who haven't dealt with
their own personal need to control the research and the
outcome, were more fearful and challenged the things I knew
were happening to me, as a direct result of being in Chiropractic care! If these professionals choose to adhere to the old
way of strict doctor/patient relationships, they may become

a vanishing species, as we as patients, change and become more informed. The life process of change takes time, but change is inevitable.

For years, as parents, we have cried out for nutritional information to use as preventive medicine, to help us keep our families healthy. It has been slow in coming, but it certainly is here now and we have plenty of choices. Another really hopeful example of this is the issue of cigarette smoking in America and the changes in attitude toward this over the past fifteen years.

In recent years, as our last two children became strong athletes, the "quick fix" to cover up the symptoms, so that they could at least perform, again took me over. Was I brainwashed or too busy to realize it or even do my own homework?

Fortunately, they were both relatively healthy, so that these prescription drugs were not needed too often. Still it again became the pattern for me.

My dependence on medicine was evident, compounded by my fear of being ill. It was as if illness was not a natural process created to rid the body of some intruder that belonged elsewhere.

I remember the children saying at that time that they didn't want to go to the doctor to get a prescription. It seemed to make them sicker. Such wisdom! It was in our son's senior year that he began to go to the chiropractor who had volunteered to help correct the injuries of the athletes at his high school.

In the previous year, as I tried to exercise with my asthma attacks, I again began moving into the world of acceptance and dependency! My parents had just died and I was feeling so drained. I did not have the patience to wait.

Under my new system with Chiropractic care, it was already late fall when I noticed that my usual change of season ailments were not coming around. I did not miss them. My husband and our children, now young adults in college, noticed the same. I was told this would happen, as I regained more balance in my body.

Twice in the last winter I had a violent allergic reaction at home to some fresh paints and my sinuses were draining profusely. By then I had become an outside observer of my body's ability to heal itself, so I was going to watch and see how it did without an antihistamine. It was fascinating, but I weakened in the final hour and took the medication because I had to go out that evening. That was the first time.

The second time I was going to be a little braver. Now we are only talking about one antihistamine pill. This was two months later and even with wearing a professional ventilation mask, the fumes of the paint stripper I was using got to me again. This time I made up my mind that I would weather the storm. I was surprised at my own preoccupation with all of this.

I could choose to relieve my discomfort with medication, or I could let my body naturally do the healing. I stayed objective. I really was having difficulty with this one, but I wanted to learn the lesson I used to know when I was a child. Then, we did not run to the doctor even though office visits were only $3.50 a visit. This wasn't that long ago - especially now that I am feeling fifteen years younger!

I, actually, felt that I needed a twelve-step program. I'll tell you, though, when I didn't take the medicine and my body healed the draining sinuses on its own in two days, I was very aware of the clarity I felt through the whole experience. I had not felt sick and did not have that groggy side effect that comes with the medicines. It was a simple experiment that effectively made a big difference to me.

Since the winter before I began Chiropractic care a year and a half ago, I have not used or needed my inhaler. I have also thrown out all of the antihistamines and other "self-help" over the counter medications.

I later found out that the professional mask I used only had a dust filter and was not the charcoal filtered type to protect me from the poisons in the paint stripper! Oh the wonderful healing powers of this magnificent creation called the human body!

In recent years I had literally become immune to the effect most aspirin-type medications had on my headaches. They did not work anymore. Now a year and a half later my headaches are just about gone and so is my dependency on aspirin!

So often even simple medications have so many side effects that we never really know what is the true illness or the symptom due to the drug medication. Doing our homework and asking the right questions is very important for our good health.

This is my story. Each of us have to make our own decisions on what we should and should not try. A long time has passed, since I took that chance and I like the results. This has been a healthy year - healthy in mindbodyspirit. Those in my family who have also been in Chiropractic care, have had no need for any medication. I was told this might happen and I liked it!

I took a doctor break! I went to the beach for a week on Long Island and spent quiet moments reflecting. Things were still okay. I was beginning to understand the process. At this point I had been in chiropractic care for only a few months, but I could definitely feel a difference physically. It was a healthy difference!

CHAPTER SEVEN

The Partnership Of Trust:
Your Signature Story

Sometimes it is difficult to explain the intuitive response inside you that says you can trust someone. It may have something to do with the positive energy you feel in the room with that person, or the freedom created by non-judgment. You just know that there exists a certain integrity that projects a sense of wholeness and unconditional love.

Even more powerful sometimes is the effect created by someone's personal story - a story that has led that person to this place in time. A "signature story," as it is called, is uniquely owned. It is part of a persons biography.

When you share your story with others, you become very real to those who listen. It is a full body experience that involves all the senses and expresses that part of you that makes you approachable and, maybe, even vulnerable. It's always easier to tell someone else's story, but it is your personal story that holds the power.

Most of us were raised to believe that vulnerability makes us weak. On the contrary, after many years of working with young people and adults, and as a mother, teacher, and group facilitator, I have learned that it is from our vulnerability that we gain our strength and bring people towards us.

For some of us, showing our human side is difficult. When our protective walls are up, we become unapproachable. When we share our stories, others become close to us and offer support. This often invites the listener to express their personal story without fear of judgment.

This sharing gives us a chance to see and understand the universality of our feelings. It fosters security and hope in that we are not alone. This describes the support group experience which can be brought into any of our relationships. Here we find the safety of unconditional love and support.

When I told my doctor in an earlier visit, how some of the recent events in my life had caused me to face my own mortality, he told me that several years ago he too had a similar experience. This greatly affected him causing him to become more focused on his purpose and mission in life and to connect spiritually with his work and his patients.

It was his signature story that told me that his work was connected to his faith in God. That was all I needed to know, for him to earn my trust and loyalty – that and the fact that he said he could fix my neck! These two things became the foundation for my trust.

It is part of the mystery unfolding, or the spiritual connection that occurs when people share their life stories with one another.

When creating your own signature story:
- let it be free flowing and honest
- speak slowly and keep your heart connected to the words
- share your confusion and sense of powerlessness
- be vulnerable about the joys and fears you experience at the time of the story

- describe your moments of truth that give you hope and empower you towards fulfilling your purpose and mission in life
- explain how this experience affected your life and the lessons you learn from it.

I had to give the healing process time, whether I wanted to or not. Very often, without my telling the doctor anything, he would go right to the point of a recent injury during the adjustment. In the doctor's office I was never judged no matter what I said or how I said it. This was good! In the beginning I had a lot to say, as I learned to listen in silence!

I came to understand him to be a person who was so focused on what he did that what we said as patients, very often seemed irrelevant, especially, if we talked symptoms. I had a lot of difficulty understanding this at first. To let go of this was an interesting challenge.

This insecurity and lack of verbal reassurance created many self-defeating behaviors on my part, as a patient. I was still focusing on the symptoms instead of recognizing that this was a slow process of change toward a new way of thinking.

Illness, injury and emotional crisis often forces us to be vulnerable, controlled by our feelings of dependency and helplessness. We humans do not like that. We try to hold back and cover it up, rather than acknowledge it. My injury was something I could not visualize, since I did not have the understanding of my own transitions through the process. Until I could learn to completely trust the intuitive process of healing, I needed simple affirmations to give me hope. When you don't see the whole picture, you tend to feel victimized.

Hope is created together, within the partnership, and provides the affirmation, security and reassurance that is so vital to the healing process.

A true partnership requires communication and mutual respect. It is also not a relationship if one party does all the talking or does all the giving without any input from the other person. There must also be an acknowledgment of the feelings and concerns of one another for it to be a healthy relationship.

When we withhold information from patients who really need it, no matter how insignificant we may think it is, we rob them of hope. This can actually become a form of abuse. Many of us have experienced broken promises and shattered dreams in our lives. This lack of reassurance is unfair and not comfortable. It needs to be addressed and understood as damaging. Accountability for this behavior is important.

I truly believe that people who are exhausted, burned out and hurting or who deny their own feelings, hurt others because no one, in their view, seems to care or listens to them. Their feelings have been stifled for so long that it is easier to just shut down, put the walls up and do the mechanical things that are part of the job. "Fix me, Doc, but don't touch me!" says the patient who denies emotional or spiritual incompleteness and who only understands the process of healing the physical injury.

Personal relationships do not always happen with individuals who find it necessary to maintain a strict "doctor/patient" relationship. This is often part of the discomfort and confusion we feel as we take the risk to change and become more open. We don't know quite how to do it, so we switch back and forth as we begin to change our behavior.

As we move beyond our own comfort zone to accept change, we may stay for a while and then get scared and pull back behind our protective walls. When we feel secure again, we will repeat the cycle. We only accept the relationship as long as we are not confused by the new guidelines.

When both things happen at once, the sensitivity to those around you and the walls of fear moving up and down, it is confusing to both the patient and the doctor. Time can be an imposing factor and staying focused on the service at hand can be another. It took me a while to understand this as being part of the process of change.

> **It is also important to make sure that patients are not forced into the role of "grateful children" who override their feelings because of gratitude. This can only become self-defeating in the healing process.**

No one lives "rent free" in my head any more, but when communication is shut off, conversations go inward. This may result in an internal anger which, if not expressed, may "eat holes" in the weakest organ of our body. Abuse comes into our lives in many forms, whether we like it or not. This is so unnecessary and sometimes so automatic that the behavior is not connected to the intention.

The solution to this is not about confrontation. It's about awareness. We let it happen when we cannot identify our inner strength to set our boundaries and make it stop. Just to be able to say, "I will no longer allow that kind of behavior to be part of my life," or, simply put, "that response is no longer acceptable," releases that inner strength and sense of pride that comes when we choose to no longer be manipulated by others. Abuse hides behind many masks, whether we are conscious of them or not.

> **In the world today a major paradigm shift is taking place from one model, where there is control or power over another person, (secrets reign) to another model that has shared power with ownership and input from others (collaboration).**

Within the new model, communication is the necessary element for success. So many of us come from the control model. We grew up in that system. We studied under it and maybe even rebelled against it! Subconsciously, until we become aware of the effect this shift has on the patients' healing process, it will be difficult, if not impossible, for them to take responsibility for their own knowledge and education concerning their illness or injury.

When people are controlled or oppressed, no one ever has to worry about their behavior. They follow directions and do what they are told. But oppression forces people out of esteem. They do not see their choices and they lose their identity, since their identity now becomes what others want of them. Their "fight or flight" survival needs and their feelings of being trapped causes them to behave in a predictable way, like a caged wild animal. Due to their misbehavior we can then get others to judge them as bad.

If we allow individuals to become participants in the decision-making process, we let them know that they are valued, as intelligent and contributing human beings. Who they are and what they do makes a difference.

Empowerment takes place when they make the decision to take the risk to change themselves. They take full responsibility for the outcome of their life process, no longer expecting others to do it for them.

The road blocks that have inhibited their personal and professional growth can then be removed. They can then choose to become all that they were meant to be.

When individuals have choices and take ownership of their attitudes and behaviors, they then can begin to see others as allies and resources for new knowledge. As they let go of their resistance to others, they can create win/win situations that build positive healing relationships through better communication.

When a person feels good about themselves, they can begin to feel good about others. They become less judgmental and controlling and more accepting of the differences they see in others.

Avoidance of confrontation at all costs does not give a person the room they need to be honest with themselves.

The challenge is to let go of what locks you into old behaviors and takes you away from being your true self. You do care and you do have choices to take that risk to open up and say what you're thinking without fear of the anger this may provoke. The following strategies from my book, *Does Anyone Hear Our Cries For Help?* assists individuals in accepting those things in life that cannot be changed.

Strategies For Successful Detachment

1. Decide not to be a victim
2. Identify the problem and understand who owns it.
3. Separate from the problem and do not own it, unless you are part of the problem.
4. Acknowledge that we are powerless over another's choice of behavior.
5. Let go of what we cannot control. We can only change ourselves.
6. Set clear boundaries for certain behaviors
7. Provide reasonable, achievable consequences for any violation of those boundaries.
8. Follow-through with these consequences.
9. Change your reaction to their behavior, so others can alter their behavior.
10. Work on healthy detachment with love by taking care of yourself.
11. Practice, practice, practice so that others can no longer push your buttons.

CHAPTER EIGHT

My Fear Of Dependency

There was a good reason for all this turmoil inside of me. It goes back to the fact that I was having great difficulty being a patient. I did not want to feel that I had to be there in this doctor's care in order to be healed, or to have my pain relieved. I felt trapped by a system I did not understand. I never expected to revisit those feelings of co-dependency that I thought I had successfully let go of years ago. These old emotions were building up within me. I did not like being out of control and at the same time feeling controlled.

I knew that I needed extra support as the pressure on the cells of my neck was being released and creating an emotional upheaval within me.

My feelings of discomfort and confusion were every-where and I had no idea where they were coming from. I felt so out of control. I took responsibility for what was inside of me, but I also wondered, if I were asking too many questions? The questions just would not go away. I relaxed and learned to let go again and again, and trusted that there was a lesson in this for me - somewhere.

It was so difficult to focus on my own needs. It was always more rewarding to help others. I had forgotten to love myself and to replenish my energy! I could no longer stuff my feelings and keep quiet about my truth. My mind, body and spirit were crying out for help! Everything inside me seemed to be at war.

The feelings of being trapped were coming back to me and centering in my neck and upper back. I was very uncomfortable and frustrated and in much pain.

For some reason I was also beginning to feel that I was back in the nineteen seventies. As a premed major in college, I was from the generation that affirmed the importance of a strict doctor/patient relationship. In those years this had been protocol, greatly encouraged within the medical profession. Doctors feared that if they became too involved with their patients, somehow, something might be lost. Involvement required risk taking, flexibility and boundaries, but not control.

My experience has shown me that I do not do well with the lack of dialogue that this control model produces. When I am vulnerable and in pain, the last thing I need is to go to a doctor with body language that expresses "power over" me.

If Chiropractic care is holistic in its approach to mindbodyspirit, and I believe it is, then to me this non-responsiveness to patient input is a conflict in terms. What a patient says cannot be negated or ignored.

This was uncomfortable for me. Actually, it was my misinterpretation. What was happening in me was a different kind of healing, one that had a different set of guidelines. I still wanted to talk symptoms and pain because that was what I was used to.

My discomfort was inside of me and not necessarily done to me. Chiropractic care is a way of life, as I was to come to understand in time, but not just yet. I needed to stay in the present moment and remain fully committed to the process, wherever it was going to take me. In a positive way I was learning things I didn't ask for. I continued to pray for guidance and understanding.

I could not deny the power of my mind in the healing process. Attitude and contentment are so important if we are to heal properly. Depending on the individual's personality, most patients come into a doctor's office concerned about the outcome of their injury. I was one of them. I was fearful of how long it was going to take me to get back the full movement in my neck and fearful that my immobility was just part of the aging process and may never change.

> **Margaret Caudill, author of *Managing Your Pain Before It Manages You*, suggests that, "Denying or ignoring the pain allows the body and mind to suffer more because of the unacknowledged stress of the pain." When our fears are recognized, they no longer beg for attention.**

Was I asking too many questions? Special friends, involved for many years in Chiropractic care outside of this office, told me to let go. I need not overanalyze or personalize my situation. Oh well! I would try not to, but my body was changing and I needed some answers. I wanted to know what was happening inside of me. Besides, I was fascinated by the whole process.

> **I was a science teacher. Wasn't the doctor the same? Doesn't the word doctor mean teacher? Or was he to be a teacher of a different kind?**

Teachers come to us in many ways with their different gifts. Sometimes, we are unfamiliar with their methods of teaching. Yet, as we release our expectations, we can learn so much from them.

My doctor did not have a need to know the affect his care had on his patients. I could feel his confidence. He had twenty-five years experience and knew what he was doing. He had no idea how important this information had become to me. This just made me more inquisitive!

But then, maybe this doctor knew something I didn't know. Wasn't that the reason I came to him in the first place?

Wasn't he there to facilitate a healing he said he could do? Isn't that the reason any one of my healers, helpers, wizards and guides have come into my life - to give me something I didn't know I needed?

What is my responsibility, as a patient and what is the doctor's? Am I to research my own disease or injury? Is it in my expectation of what I think my care should be that I fall short, as a patient? Do my fears inhibit the healing process?

Sometimes the most difficult part is to get past the fear of intimidation and to know that we have a right to ask for what we need. It is so much easier to blame others for what we will not do for ourselves.

How can I expect anyone to know my questions, or even to have the answers, if I don't ask them? And if true healing is a mystery unfolding in its own time, aren't there always going to be questions that cannot be answered at the moment? Was life just one big question?

Taking responsibility to research our own injury or illness no matter how intimidated we may feel will help us be better patients. The resources are there to build our confidence in knowing that we are not alone. At the time I just did not know what I needed to know. I was too caught up in the physical changes in my body and looking for logical explanations. I had not let go of my fears.

The more we, as patients, know about our own health and well being, the less we will be dependent on others for the answers to our questions. When we share in this responsibility, we become our own advocates for our own good health. My search for knowledge was directed toward fulfilling my need for inner peace. This took my healing far beyond just the effects produced by an injured neck. I wanted to eliminate these fears.

I have been asked several times why I stayed in Chiropractic care, especially, when all my old co-dependency issues began to surface. The reason was simple. I wanted to take responsibility for my own feelings and not blame anyone else for them. Also, I was very curious as to how all this applied to other relationships in my life.

My challenge, as a patient, was to know and to truly believe that it was time to focus on me and my own healing and to let go of my need to "rescue" others. I wanted my good health back. If this was how I had to get it, then this was how it had to be. No one else could do it for me.

Why wouldn't any helping professional be affected by co-dependent issues? Many have highly developed intuitive senses that allow them to read body language. It becomes part of their job to know and understand what is going on with their patients, clients, students or employees.

Some dependency is necessary in the beginning. The practitioner has the knowledge. The patient/client needs this knowledge to understand and overcome their fear of the unknown. Once this initial need for help is acknowledged, patients then can make a personal commitment to actively participate in their own healing journey. This is an important beginning.

Still believing that the answers had to come from outside of me, I did not realize that all I ever needed to know could be found in silence from within, if I could only silence myself! I was working on it! Centering helped, but it didn't last. I had to learn to practice being quiet at other times in my life.

Even with all the incongruities that I sensed everywhere, I still found an incredible peacefulness in the silence within the adjustment room of the doctor's office. He used pressure points, unconditional love and a lot of positive energy - a nice combination. It was like an oasis in my life - a place where I could stop even for ten minutes in silence and evaluate my priorities and sense of purpose.

My hope was that in time I would be able to take this peacefulness out with me into my world. Eventually, this goal became so important to me that this special time for silence became a necessary part of my day.

CHAPTER NINE

Co-dependency Surrounds Me

My pain was not simple, but complex. The physical pain was obvious, but the emotional attachments came as a big surprise to me. I knew that identifying my pain and working my way through it was part of the process of change.

My experiences opened me up to a new understanding of my world at different levels - physically, emotionally, mentally and spiritually. They were all tied to a number of causes that included family life adjustments, things that limited my viewpoint and new ideas that stretched me beyond my comfort zone and forced me to either accept the changes that were asked of me let go of the issues that troubled me, or change my attitude toward them.

What I did not understand and unfortunately, it affected me greatly, was that somehow I was to ignore my pain and not talk about it unless it was screaming at me. It was like telling a person not to think about pink elephants. It doesn't work! The mind does not understand the word, "not." All I could "see" was my pain!

What I was feeling was much bigger than just the physical effects of the adjustments on my body. I began to understand that my pain was far greater than just my crooked neck. What did I know? So much was left unexplained. Finally, after three and a half months with office visits three times a week, I rebelled internally. I was living proof of the statement, "What a man thinketh in his heart, so he is."

I could not escape from it. After weeks of stifling so many feelings due to time limitation and my fear of pushing the system, I wrote the following straight from my heart:

"I came in need of chiropractic care. I came as a believer. I came because I chose to take care of me. I understood the roller coaster ride. I began the adventure.

I came as a believer with my heart and spirit wide open to give or receive. I received and observed with my eyes closed and my heart open and felt the process of healing. I felt the energy of those around me both good and not so good. I could see what others could not see. I stayed silent and focused.

I thought I understood my injury. I did not. I did not know that I did not know. The good news was that it could be fixed. I thought I asked the right questions and did the right exercises. No one ever asked me what I understood. They didn't need to. I thought I understood.

I got confused with the directions, and was afraid to ask that they be repeated. In my discomfort I forgot things quickly or half listened. People dealing with change do that often.

Good things were happening and I was feeling more balanced and strong. I thought I understood. I believed I had to in order to visualize the healing process, a process that would take time. I still did not understand.

The headaches became more intense and lasted longer. The stiffness in my neck did not go away. I understood the process. I did not understand the injury. Each visit I would recite my 'shopping list' of where it hurt. This became automatic as part of the routine, but I received no feedback.

My awareness of my injury increased. Six to eight hours of my day was consumed by this awareness. I did not stop doing the things I had always done. I stayed focused on the prevention of further injury and on the healing process.

I was not angry. I was just confused. I stayed in the present moment and let go of what I could not control. I came as a believer with my heart and spirit wide open and that has never changed.

I felt sucked in and captured by my own thoughts. Sometimes I would move the thoughts away and sometimes I allowed them to stay and visit for a while.

I felt dependent and uninformed - not sure of what questions to ask. I had forgotten most of the early directions for special exercises. This didn't seem to matter since no one ever mentioned them again. I was given new ones.

I could pretend that there was no progress. How would I know? There is so much silence. Those thoughts I easily dropped, since they would do me no good.

Everything in my life affirmed my belief that we tend to become what we feel we are. My preoccupation with the intensity of this commitment to heal what I did not fully understand had become an internal conflict. I felt no empowerment.

For ten years I intensely climbed out of the pit that kept me in this self-defeating thinking pattern. I know the techniques, but the basic philosophy of chiropractic care I feel through my lack of knowledge is in conflict with these techniques.

I must remain dependent on or co-dependent with the Chiropractor or the system in order to acquire good health. "Co-dependency is a terminal illness." -

(Melody Beattie: *Co-dependent No More.*) Is it part of the process? I don't want to go there. My only other choice is not to continue the process - a choice I won't even consider because I understand and trust the physical aspects.

Where is the empowerment to learn to care for oneself? Where is the personal growth? What is the connection? Why am I so tired when I'm again doing everything right?

I know the answer, but do other patients know the answer too? Are their feelings the same as mine? Are we all guarding the same secret? Can they too feel the aura of co-dependency around them?

Here I am again, preoccupied with my own personal choice and challenge. Here I am again with a smile on my face saying I'm fine, fine, fine!

I am not fine. My mind and body are in conflict. One cannot heal when this is happening. The answer cannot come without communication.

I thought I understood. I tried to explain it. Blind faith does not work to my advantage. I came as a believer and that never changed. Maybe I need more than that. Is anyone else crying for help? Great title for a book!!"

As I share this, I take full ownership for the way I was feeling when I wrote it. Feelings are neither right or wrong. They are just feelings. I was beginning to revisit my own issues of co-dependency to a system that was actually giving me an opportunity for such special care from a doctor whose gifts to correct and heal went far beyond the issues. Later on, I learned that the doctor was fully unaware of these frustrations in me.

Most people do not recognize the impact of co-dependent issues on their own lives or within their environment until it is brought to their attention.

Awareness is always the first step to understanding its influence on everyone. Since everything seems normal to what always has been, individuals often have difficulty knowing what to do with the information after they receive it.

My fear of dependency on the doctor came from my own belief, or I should say, old tape, that he was the expert and, therefore, the one who should be telling me what to do and how to do it, in order for me to get better. Why wouldn't I believe this? Isn't this why we ask to be in the care of this doctor? Who was there to tell me otherwise? Isn't this the traditional way? What was it that I was looking for? There seemed to be no logical explanation.

I honestly believe that when we constantly accommodate the needs and wishes of others, we lose our own identity and ability to think for ourselves. We will no longer bother to trust our instincts and perceptions. When other people do our thinking for us, it erodes our self-esteem and robs us of that balance in mindbodyspirit that we seek to reclaim.

This was my internal conflict. I felt no empowerment to seek out the answers to my own questions. I did not like how that felt. By not forcing the issue, which for me was the lack of mutual dialogue with the doctor, I was enabling that behavior to continue. I could not change anything at the moment, so instead, I let go of it and learned a different lesson. I did not want to risk being anyone's conscience. I did not want to be the voice of change for someone else. Besides, these were my perceptions.

"People can be hated for no other reason than because they impersonate conscience."
                                                Lady Baron

I was feeling better. The physical pain in my neck and shoulders had not gone away and the movement in the neck was still limited, but many other good things were happening. All I wanted was to be a good patient, so I could feel better and get on with my life. I knew I could be a good patient and do what I was told! I had always been the "peacemaker" and the "perfect child" in my home growing up. Why wouldn't I also want to be the perfect patient?

Somehow, I felt the system was holding me in bondage. I also knew I was letting it happen, since I chose to be there! As Stephen Covey says in his book, *The Seven Habits of Highly Effective People,* "Our ultimate freedom is our internal power to express options."

I could not see my choices through my physical and emotional pain. I did not want to quit until this all went away. I wanted so much to trust the system and the facilitator of my care.

My own recovery process from co-dependency, taught me that it was very important that I do the following:
   • Think for myself and be who I am
   • Give only what I really want to give
   • Hold on tight to my integrity and beliefs
   • Do only what I have time to do
   • Think positively and with a clear head
   • Let go of compromising relationships
   • Never permit others to drain energy from me
   • Seek inner peace and good health without guilt
   • Live life to the fullest

Although I did not like being a patient, the adjustment room became "sacred space," where I sorted things out and made myself accountable to whatever goal I set for that week. I knew that I did not cause the situations in which I found myself, so I detached. I thought! I didn't have to "fix" anything but me - even though I thought I could help at the time! I tried to remember the three C's, as I heard the cries of others calling out to me:

- I did not *cause* it!
- I can't *control* it!
- I can't *cure* it!

It was good that I chose not to allow myself to shift my focus away from that of being a patient. I remained focused on my own healing. I could only do me and that was a full time job.

Even with all my detachment skills, I found it very difficult to block out the things in my life that I saw and felt were affecting me and my well being. It was so easy for me to hop on the "roller coaster of life" with whoever invited me and to go for a ride!

I kept practicing each day and every visit. Interestingly, this forced me to look at my own control issues and the expectations I had for others to behave in a certain way. Was this another lesson in letting go? I had been so well trained to hang on!

A friend of mine, another "guide," many years ago, said to me, "Did you think these issues would really go away?" At least I was willing to name them as I felt my issues of co-dependency creep in on me. They always seemed to cycle in my life. When things became too difficult, they would "make me" want to fly away.

Co-dependency is many things. For me it has always been connected to self-esteem and the loss of self. If who I am depends on what other people think of me, then who am I without their judgment?

> **If I give up who I am for the approval of someone else, then I have lost my freedom to choose my own path.**

My identity becomes lost, as it is now absorbed into the whims and controls of another person. This leads to emotional exhaustion from negative thoughts running through my brain.

> **"Burnout occurs when individuals are not permitted to care - not because they do not care. It is their mission in life to care. Let's slow down the system so these helping professionals can again care."**
>
> **Dr. Janet Quinn**

Co-dependents care so much. It is what they do to help others who may be feeling victimized and need rescuing. Of their very essence they will give and give without taking a break. As they wear out, they often feel unappreciated and misunderstood and wonder why no one helps them. Asking for help is very difficult for them, as they never want to impose on others. They fear rejection and have difficulty speaking up. When communication ends, burnout begins.

Co-dependency releases feelings similar to being pulled into an environment that surrounds them and sucks the energy out of them. They climb up the hill frantically trying to get away from these feelings, but they follow them everywhere, taking over their every moment. There is no escape.

At first this is comfortable because it feels good to care. But when no one appreciates their generosity and sensitivity, these bottled up emotions become a complete distraction. The only escape is to stay away, separating oneself from the input of this energy. If they remain they learn to detach by changing their attitude toward what is capturing them and let go of their need to control that which is out of their control. This is a choice. They can also turn it over to their God or their Higher Power to handle for them, over and over again, until they really get it!

"If I can step aside and let God's will be done, I free myself from anxiety and a mistaken sense of responsibility."

Carl Jung

I was definitely practicing letting go of what I could not control - the feelings and behaviors of those outside of me - every day! This was a wonderful lesson for me and never an easy one. I wanted to remain sensitive to their feelings, knowing that I did not have to own them. This personal challenge became a very powerful part of my healing journey. It tested my ability to stay focused on being a patient, and to let go of my own issues of control.

Let Go…and Let God

As children bring their broken toys with
tears for us to mend, I brought my broken
dreams to God, because He was my friend.

But then, instead of leaving Him in peace to
work alone, I hung around and tried to
help, with ways that were my own.

At last, I snatched them back and cried,
how can you be so slow?"

"My child," He said, "What could I do? You
never did let go!"

Author Unknown

CHAPTER TEN

The Spirituality Of Healing: Listening In Silence

Questions continued to run through my head out of control. I analyzed them again and again. I wasn't sure what I was supposed to do with them. There never seemed to be enough time to have them answered.

Mostly because of my own internal resistance, I chose not to ask the questions out loud. When I did, they were always answered; but I felt so rushed and limited by my fear of cutting into the time of the next patient that I held back. Again I was worrying about other people. It was so easy for me to do this.

Even though I was feeling trapped by the slowness of my healing progress, I maintained my commitment to keep on going. Many things were better, but there seemed to be no end in sight. I needed some hope.

I decided to pray - really pray. "Dear God, teach me to trust your timing." I still wanted my timing!

All my life I have been one of those people who had great conversations with God. I just didn't tell anyone. One of my earliest memories of these discussions happened when I was in third grade. I had cheated on a test, and I was so frightened that I had committed a mortal sin that God and I had this talk! I looked it up in my "Bible," *The Baltimore Catechism*, and found out that in order for a sin to be mortal I had to know that it was and do it anyway! Imagine! I was eight years old. Well, that wasn't good enough. I didn't know if I knew, so I made a deal with God. I told him I needed a sign. If it rained tomorrow, then I would know that I did not commit a mortal sin. It rained!

There were many times in my angry years that I would have open discussions with God in my head for hours. I wore myself out with my control issues and my "if only they would change" issues. I could not listen very well in those days. It was a one sided conversation. God is patient.

Today I take full responsibility for what thoughts I will allow and not allow in my head. These questions now were a different story. I was not angry toward any one person. I was more angry at the system that stimulated these responses in me. I refused to entertain any feelings of anger toward someone who could not fulfill my expectations or who did not do something the way I though they should. I felt gratitude and appreciation for the many good things that were happening physically to my body. These offset my feelings of emotional discomfort that I was still trying to understand.

Dr. John DeMartini's in his book, *Count Your Blessings*, tells us that it is impossible to be grateful and angry at the same time. He is right.

I did not like the control my thoughts had over my body. When I held my feelings back, my tension headaches came back. If I felt the stress of this dishonesty with myself, then my neck and shoulder muscles hurt.

What did I know? This whole process was different from anything I had ever experienced. I paid attention to the physical positions of my posture to avoid over stressing the muscles of my neck and back. I also used the time to set my priorities enforcing my boundaries, eating properly, exercising, reading, interacting with others, listening to tapes, letting go of the need for medicines.

I stayed focused on these choices for my own spiritual, physiological and psychological well being. I was very aware of how my mental attitude affected the pain in my body. If I held back my feelings, then my tension headaches became worse. This was quite powerful.

With all my questions calling out for answers, I created my own internal Spirit Guide "meditatively released from my subconscious." as Bernie Siegel describes in his book, *Love, Medicine and Miracles.* **"I found my guide to be spontaneous, aware of my feelings and an excellent advisor."**

My Guide and I became good friends. Some people call this their angel, or Spirit Guide, or the God within. To me the name doesn't matter. As far back as I can remember, I always felt that I was having these discussions with my God. First, a question would come into my mind and I would think about it. Then we would silently talk. When I was through, as soon as I got the answer from within my soul, I was able to let go of the question. There were even questions answered that I never asked, but needed the answers.

No longer did I need to depend on others to sort out these changes. I was moving to a different level of understanding. My dependency wasn't working anyhow! This sounds strange, but in some ways I became my own therapist. Why not! I knew all the techniques!

My life became one big prayer. This whole healing process was so much bigger than me. My Spirit Guide helped me with this. Prayer taught me to let go of where this journey was leading me.

I accepted everything that crossed my path, as something that had a meaningful purpose connected to my healing journey. Every experience, every person, every conversation, every author, I believed, added something.

These were truly my healers, helpers, wizards and guides along my path. This approach also replaced some of the sadness I was feeling with love. I began to understand love as the natural frequency around me and feel that I could handle whatever was happening and that this all had meaning for me yet to discover.

The Power of Prayer

1. Bring into your awareness the desire to connect with God
2. Keep your prayer conversational and let go of the rules
3. Choose words that empower a relationship with God
4. Pray for the highest good of all
5. Incorporate it into your life
6. Surrender your will and transform it into God's will
7. Release the need to control every moment
8. Place all you do in God's hands to achieve harmony in mindbodyspirit
9. Open your heart to see God in everyone.
10. Be grateful for all that is good in your life

My goals for eating properly and exercising were helping me physically feel so much better. My energy was definitely coming back, although I continued to feel trapped and aware of the situations around me that I could not influence.

I stayed in the present moment realizing how my healing process would be affected if I did not detach. It was so easy for me to regress into old patterns, when I felt closed in and vulnerable in my pain.

I was careful not to ask too many questions. I was careful not to take too much time from other patients. I was careful not to offend anyone. I was careful not to break any of the egg shells I was walking on!!

This was not good. I was beginning to recognize that I was feeling entrapped, caged and closed in by my own issues of emotional abuse. Time had become the control over me. I was not relaxed, yet I was able to relax for the adjustment most of the time. If I didn't, the doctor caught me and brought this to my attention! Gently, I chose again to trust the process and the "facilitator" completely. Headaches, chronic pain and emotional upheaval all came with the package, as the nerve pressure was being released.

I was definitely having difficulty accepting my role as a patient especially now that my co-dependency issues were beginning to resurface. Where was all this coming from? I thought I only had a crooked neck that needed fixing!

This whole process of healing and what I was learning from it was taking up residency in my head. What was going on here? At one point I felt so trapped in my dependency on the doctor for my healing that I felt totally consumed, and unable to separate the two and could not move it out. I was so preoccupied that I was losing sight of my responsibility for all this.

I remembered my dream and my dad's encouragement. "Everything would be all right, Baby." I stayed connected to that loving thought.

I also knew that the only way past all this emotional baggage was to take the risk to go through it. Wasn't that the whole purpose in being here: to bring the mind, body and spirit into balance? My neck injury was only the vehicle to get me there.

"Spirituality is a journey within. The soul at peace is the one who knows the healing. To seek

so that we can then live in Faith. This comes with
being still, listening and trusting that this peace
can heal broken lives."

Rev. Dr. Nancy J. Lane

My soul was not at peace. Father Jim O'Brien, S.J., a dear
friend and my spiritual advisor, since my college days,
suggested that I go within and just listen. What a thought: to
go inside in silence and listen. He has been such a special
support person for me along this journey. He has listened to
my questions, heard my stories and watched me grow,
affirming every moment.

Quietly I sat in silence and went inside in the true sense
of the word and prayed to see what was immobilizing me.
Again, I found that it was my need to control that which I
could not control. I made the conscious decision to replace
my need to control with the desire to love unconditionally
those whom I thought I might want to change and to respond
out of love and not resistance. "All I could do is love them," I
would tell myself. I practiced and practiced this, week after
week, until I saw the effect it had on my response to others
and their response to me. It transformed my life as I will
explain later.

I had so many rules for how things should be without
any point of reference for my attitude. Each visit, one by one,
I was being dismantled. So often, I felt like a horse whose
spirit was being broken - taken apart bit by bit and later to be
rebuilt with stronger and better parts. I was losing myself
and compromising my beliefs in what I was experiencing.
Everything hurt: my mind, my body and my spirit.

"The power of God is life giving. Healing is
painful. God will take apart everything in our
body and soul and put it back together in a new
order. To let go and trust and to live in faith
moves us away from dis-ease."

Rev. Dr. Nancy J. Lane

I felt this was happening to me. I knew that healing is never predictable even though I wanted so much to predict the outcome. I had decided from the very beginning to use this time in the Chiropractic care face down on the adjustment table as an enforced meditation retreat. It was what kept me coming in for my appointments. Even though my office visits were such brief moments, each time I chose to go within, quietly centering myself and praying for the guidance of the doctor's healing hands.

> **I continued to clear my head and connect with the doctor's intention to heal, knowing full well that his healing hands were reaching out with a willingness in silence to guide and support me through my fears. This was unspoken but definitely present in his essence.**

My neck injury was the doorway for this healing, facilitated in silence by my doctor. My mindbodyspirit with its wisdom to heal itself knows the best path for me on this journey. It has the ability to hear that inner voice that directs me, as I choose to surrender control.

> **Was it my insecurity and lack of faith in this ability to access my inner knowledge that caused me to need affirmation of my every thought? In time, I came to understand this, but not yet, and not before I faced my fears.**

The journey into silence was such a difficult one for me. I feared silence. I was afraid of what it might expose me to. In some ways I have spent my life addicted to the noise. The radio always had to be on with music playing that connected me to my emotions. I also came from a big family and spent much of my life working with young people who were seldom quiet!

In my life it was so foreign to me that it took me some time to accept it. Until I could understand it as I do now, silence did not give me anything. I never went deep enough into it to find that inner peace. I've always known somehow, that underwater when I snorkeled, there was a silence that I loved and craved. I always swim with a face mask, snorkels and fins. My family believes I'm half fish. The truth is, I'm a marine biologist and I am fearless in that silence because I feel safe. Before this moment I have never made the connection.

Is this part of my journey back to self that brings that balance into my life that I am seeking? The fish feel my peacefulness and come to me. I swim a lot and love to communicate with anything that lives underwater in the ocean and the Great Lakes. I spend time in both worlds. It is one of my places to which I escape.

Was this experience also part of the mind, body, spirit connection within the healing process? Is this the definition of Spirituality, that Father Leo Booth speaks about when he says, "Spirituality is how you connect to yourself and the world, mentally, emotionally and physically?"

Staying peaceful in silence has become very important to me. At first, I did not realize its power, but once I experienced its affect on my life, I wanted more and more of it.

When I feel resistance building within me, I focus on releasing those anxieties and any negativity within me. I would then do the following:
1. Relax and become centered
2. Breathe deeply several times with a cleansing breath
3. Spontaneously feel the presence of love in my life with someone whom I have a strong connection

4. Feel myself immersed in this unconditional love permeating every part of me
5. Hold on to this feeling and let it hold on to me
6. Picture the person with whom I was having difficulty
7. Transfer this unconditional love back to them removing all the imperfections thought to be present in them
8. Pray for their highest good, as God sees that to be
9. Become absorbed in the peacefulness now felt with them
10. Be grateful for this person's place in my life

I also practiced seeing God in everyone. Actually, I did this for an hour one time while riding on a train. What power and understanding it gave me! It can transform the way we all look at people and reframe our view of the world.

Traditionally, I have spent my life seeing only the inner core of goodness in people, so this approach was a little different, but the same idea. As a child, I learned very early to peel away the misbehavior of others which I judged as hurtful to arrive at this inner core. This helped me detach from (or deny) some of the incongruities of love and hate I experienced in my life with people I loved. It's like John Powell, S.J., author of *Unconditional Love* says, "there must be a pony here somewhere," as the optimistic child scrambles through a pile of horse dung!

Another area in particular along my healing journey that I wanted to look at was my healing relationship with the Catholic Church. It all fits together, as this unfolding mystery continues. I found that after the death of both my parents, I was having difficulty going to my parish church where we had raised our children for twenty years. I often joked about being a recovering Catholic. Was it connected to my co-dependency issues?

Was I feeling that I had never really been given a choice? Was I feeling controlled by the rules? What about the bumper sticker that reads, "My God is too big for one church!"

All the words I heard were so reflective of our purpose in life and death when one believes that life is about the Spiritual Journey into God. Everything that I had taken for granted before now made sense.

The concept of eternity as "life everlasting," became so real along with other truths that I thought I had understood. These realities hit me so hard that I needed a place to sort through all those years when I did not understand and only provided lip service for what I thought I knew.

"Everyday people are straying away from the church and going back to God."
Lenny Bruce

Our children, now in their twenties, were all off in their own space and time with their own spirituality. Had we really taught them the things we thought we were saying? Or was it time now for them to find the answers to their questions on their own? I was feeling sad that they could not know this wisdom that life had just taught me through this experience.

At that time I found myself angry again at those who taught me all the rules and wondered why, today, there seemed to be a new set of guidelines. I was unable to separate from my anger. I was in church for the quiet moment, to connect in community with others and to pray. Yet, there was so much "noise" in me then that my time was being spent mentally, somewhere else.

I also felt as if the priest were not saying the things that I thought I needed to hear. Even if he were, I could no longer listen. The choir that I use to love reflected "rules" I could no longer follow. I wanted to sing, but I didn't want to practice. Although permission was given to me to do it my way, because I sight read well, I could not allow myself to break the rules and not spend hours in practice like everyone else.

I felt my Church had let me down, not my God, but there was something else I couldn't put my hands on. Maybe, again, there were unfulfilled promises or expectations. Certainly this was not about any one person or situation, but an overall feeling. Perhaps, It was just that I was hurting all over and not finding any comfort in my old ways of doing things. Maybe this was the real beginning of this healing journey for me.

I always had believed that if I did A-B-C and D, then E-F-G and H would follow. I did all those things right and E-F-G and H did not follow. There was so much "stuff" on my shoulders that got in the way of my "seeing" the presence of my God that I had to do something. Maybe this was because I thought I had to look outside of myself for that God and couldn't get there because my vision was so cluttered with life's issues.

As the Rev. Dr. Nancy J. Lane explains in her program on *The Spirituality of Healing*, "It is important to understand our anger. It can help us reestablish our relationship with God. What makes us angry helps us to understand the core of our pain. Being angry at the injustices in our lives takes courage. It shows a strength of character that can bring us to peace and love. When we work with our anger, we learn to find its source and cause. This becomes an essential task of the spiritual journey. Anger is part of the grief cycle. We withdraw to protect ourselves from further grief."

I decided to go to another Catholic Church where I did not know anyone and found a priest who talked to my soul. I knew I was in the right place when he said:

...And we pray that the healing hands of God touch us and make us open so that in turn we can be the healing hands of God to others."
Rev. Charles Fontana

Isn't that what we're all about? I now know this change helped me with my own need for solitude along my healing journey. This was part of my coming to understand the true meaning of getting centered and going within to find a place of hope that I had not felt for years. It gave me the chance to detach from the noises that distracted me and to just be quiet and listen.

It was important for me to make that decision to change churches. I did it trusting my inner feelings. Now, the peacefulness and love I feel on Sunday morning I carry with me throughout the week. In time I will be able to return to the Church within my own community, as this healing journey continues.

CHAPTER ELEVEN

Cell Memory:
Revisiting The Past

I began to wonder, if all this emotional pain wasn't connected to cell memory the doctor had spoken of briefly during my first visit. It was important for me to stay focused on this part of the healing process of my mind and spirit that went along with this body!

Was this a cell memory experience I was going through that was so intense? I do know that for many years, now at least five or six, I have not felt this consumed by anything. I was really proud of the fact that I had learned to choose the amount of time any issue would remain in my head.

These new feelings seemed to have come from out of nowhere, building slowly during the fourth and fifth month of Chiropractic care. I had so much tension inside and outside of me. Was it the reason for all my questions?

A lot of things were now going on for me. These emotions I had not felt for years. Why was I feeling so trapped? I thought I had a handle on those feelings That wasn't why I came to this doctor's office. I just wanted my neck fixed! What was happening to me? Was this also a part of the package I didn't understand?

Do the cells of our body actually remember the feelings of the past, as the pressure on them is released? I did not like these feelings. I needed more answers. And why were my tears returning?

I felt such an incongruity in my role as a patient. Did I know too much or too little? Why was I rebelling so within myself at the thought of having to be a patient in need of so much care? I never wanted to be this dependent on anyone.

"Feelings bring back memories. Memories bring back emotions. Emotional energy is released, as we relive the experience or trauma, feel the pain and then move on to believing that we can do this!"

Michael Govan

When I first began Chiropractic care, we talked briefly about the effects of cell memory on the healing process. It made sense then. Of course our cells remember. We have over sixty trillion cells in our body. Daily, fifty million of these replicate themselves with exact perfection. A heart cell can continue to be a heart cell or a kidney cell will know that it is not to be a digestive gland.

I know cell theory and how genetic materials are passed on from generation to generation through cell division and DNA. Every cell of our body stores information which is used physically, as we repair an injury or as the body grows. Sometimes when our spine is misaligned (subluxation), it causes the cells in a particular area to get jammed up.

As the Chiropractor moves the vertebrae back into proper position, there occurs a release of the pressure off the compressed cells. My emotional memory, painful or pleasing, contained in those cells is also released. This emotional energy, possibly reflective of a painful situation, may have been bundled up for many years.

"Listen to your body. Listen to your voices inside. What are they saying? Pay attention to your body and it will give you a message. What is it telling you to do? Trust your instincts."

David Lee

What a gift we give to ourselves when we trust our instincts and believe we really know and see what we truly perceive. Once we let go of our doubts there is no going back. We just believe that we are on the right path moving forward.

Why was I revisiting places I didn't want to return to? I was listening to my body, but I did not like what I was feeling. There was an energy around me that was not good and I was being sucked into it. This was all too familiar and very uncomfortable. I was having good days and I was having bad days.

I forced myself to stay focused and in charge of me. I prayed. I agreed to continue through this and to experience whatever lesson it was to bring me. I was not alone. I let go of control over and over again. Yet, I felt so controlled by a system that had no intention of projecting that feeling upon me.

On a good day the doctor could sense my aura of positive energy. I could sense it too. He would always ask me what was going on for me that was so good. It was fun knowing he knew.

This happened twice about a month apart. Both times I had made the decision not to go back to teach full time. It would have meant a teaching position along with eligibility for retirement. I let it go. I knew I belonged in a different place. There was a purpose for all this happening in my life and its meaning was still unfolding. I was willing to wait for the answer.

The summer my parents died, I went to New York for three months to be with them. My choice had a much higher purpose and no amount of money could have bought me any more time with them. I called this self-imposed unemployment.

Even with our last two children in college, I let go believing that I was at least as important as the "lilies of the field and the birds of the air…" I had to have faith that everything was to be as it was. Money can be a very big part of our lives. It solves many problems, but we can never buy those things most precious to us.

Money

Money can buy a bed,
    but not a restful night's sleep.
Money can buy you food,
    but not fill up you hunger.
Money can buy a book,
    but not wisdom or intelligence.
Money can buy a luxury
    but not inner peace and beauty.
Money can buy a house,
    but not give you a home.
Money can buy a remedy,
    but not heal your mindbodyspirit
Money can buy acquaintances,
    but not true friendship.
Money can buy entertainment,
    but not true joyfulness
Money can buy a cemetery plot,
    but not a place in Heaven.

Others in my life were having some difficulty with this choice, but then how they felt about what I saw my purpose in life to be, was not my concern. At this point who I was did not depend on what anyone thought of me. These were tough decisions especially for those to whom they were meant. I felt that I was learning my lessons well.

In my heart I knew that it was time for me to face my fears and to speak my truth. From here on I decided to truly be myself. Each visit I practiced even for a brief moment without pretense. I wanted me back again. I liked what I was finding!

Dr. Carl A. Hammerschlag, M.D. a distinguished psychiatrist, author, storyteller and healer so clearly describes the importance of this in his writings on mind/body/spirit medicine. "Open yourself to looking at everything you thought you once knew and see it from another perspective. Change is the biological order of the universe. Welcome change. Above all do not fear. Whatever it is that frightens you, look at it straight. Otherwise it has you. You will never out run it.

Tell the truth. The gift you have to share is the truth that you are. Be the change you want to create in others. Allow them to see in you the credibility that is the richness of your talent. Touch them in ways that remind you of what you also like best in yourself and you will touch them with the gift that is your lovingness."

CHAPTER TWELVE

The Release of Energy That Healed More Than My Neck

Letting go again I became centered. I stayed focused on my healing. I was on an emotional roller coaster and did not know why. I wanted to stay anchored, but the ground was sandy and nothing would hold. The headaches became more intense. They were not explained. They were only a symptom of something else the doctor was going after, as he facilitated my healing. I was confused and remained quiet. What was this body of mine asking of me?

I was not happy. I was in enough physical pain to believe that my body had become one giant head and neck, if you can picture that! I came in to the Chiropractor four times that week. In therapy, AA or Al-anon four times in one week means that you need a lot of support to get past the rough edges that might suck you in. I knew I needed extra support and that it was safe enough to ask for it. They were all wonderful.

I could feel the confidence of the doctor. I never wavered on my trust in his ability. I knew that he had a strong spiritual connection with the God who guided his hands. I told him one time that I would love to know what his healing hands "see," as he goes through his usual routine of adjusting my spine. I found much peacefulness in that knowledge and belief.

Faith is letting go of control so far that all that is left is faith and that tells you all you need to know.

I wasn't there yet, but I was working on it. I trusted myself and believed I could do this. Everything hurt. Something was blocked and was not letting go. Was it mind, body or spirit? The doctor had been here before with other patients and understood what could not be explained. When we believe this in our heart, we know that it is the Spirit of God working through each of us that creates our special gifts. I prayed and prayed again, focused and let go. It was out of my control.

The emotional roller coaster was accelerating me forward and there was no slowing it down. There were so many tears. With my body face down on the adjustment table in the fifth month since I began my visits, I felt the tremendous surge of emotional energy break free. It was probably happening physically too. Spiritually, I could not let go any further.

I felt as if every ounce of bottled up resistance inside of me was being pulled out of me and released through the crown of my head. It was the complete opposite of being sucked in by my issues of co-dependency. It was very visual in my mind and so powerful. This was a complete release.

I felt a calmness. I knew at that moment without words much more than my neck had been healed. I had experienced something that I could not speak about for over a week.

That day and in that moment my cells remembered my feelings of entrapment and pain on the worst day of my life back fifteen years ago. It was then that I first learned my survival depended upon my taking charge of my life and setting boundaries and changing my habits that enabled uncomfortable behaviors around me to continue! It was a time in my life when I felt like a doormat, walked upon and abused, as only I could have allowed it to happen. I felt the loneliness of abandoned dreams and the emptiness that comes when we allow others to take over our lives and decide our destiny.

Following the release, all that pain was gone and with it went the headaches. My body cells had worked out their memory of that pain. It was incredible. I could move my neck further in both directions, and two months later even more mobility returned. There was such a clarity of thought within me. I immediately knew that I was no longer "climbing up hill," pretending that I was fine. It felt good to be honest.

Inside, my body energy floated around in many directions for several weeks. I eagerly wanted to understand the Chiropractic care that now had become so much a part of my life. It was definitely a new way of life for me and a new way of thinking.

I had gone off track and now I was back on track, but this was an even better track with rewards far beyond any expectation I might have ever had.

I was going to enjoy it and took all this energy with me to Mackinaw Island where I did a Pre-Conference program with the Michigan Counselors Association. I was flying high with my feet planted firmly on the ground, a ground that was no longer made of sand. Out of fairness to my audience I actually had to be careful not to be overly energetic.

Having read the Celestine Prophecy by James Redfield several times that summer, I felt like I had experienced all nine insights at once. In fact when I asked some friends that weekend to tell me about his book, The Tenth Insight, which at the time I had not yet read, in unison they said to me, "We cannot tell you because you have to experience it yourself!" For those of you who have read the book, you know that was a "Gotcha!"

None of my energy stayed in one place. It was much like a game my body was playing with itself. The energy bounced all over everywhere. I had been told by my doctor that I would probably notice that I did not need as much sleep as I had previously, but who was counting.

The doctor was right. I would wake up in the night, ready to start my day only three hours after I went to sleep. It was so new to me and I felt so good that I would get up and sleep later when I was tired. Only, I wasn't tired by my old standards. I, actually, liked the guy who said, "If we didn't have any clocks, we would never age!" That sounded good to me.

This new experience was a true gift of time. What a present: two extra hours a day was added to my life and a year later this has not changed!

When you think of the possibilities of what this all means to one's health and well being, you can begin to ask the question: Who is the healer? Who is the facilitator? Is this really connected to Chiropractic care? I would have to tell you that at this point I am a believer, but I'm not done yet! Could there really be any more?

I still did not want to have all these visits to the doctor's office, but I wanted all the positive healthy results and now I really trusted the system no matter what I was feeling – trapped by the system or free with energy bouncing in every direction inside of me. I still didn't understand it.

I will go on! Why did I feel such an incongruity of role? What was happening? I wrote the following as a stream of consciousness one month later. It was the day after I had taken the courage to ask the doctor two month's worth of questions within about fifteen minutes.

"I am still a believer, but something is not right! My energy is exploding with no place to go. Nothing inside of me seems centered. I have so many questions. I would wear anyone out, if I even began to ask them. My perception says that I am not in the right place to ask them. So I am silent again giving into the will of those around me in a process predetermined by years of experience.

My REM sleep is all messed up. Instead of cycling back to sleep after three or four hours, I wake up wired with this explosion of all the self-contained energy locked up inside me from a thirty year injury to my neck. I am running. I am walking, teaching and speaking. I am excited that all five children will be home this weekend, together for the first time in two years.

Do I have to go back again and learn to let go of what I cannot control - the convictions, determinations and behaviors of those around me? Is it right to believe that these behaviors make me think that I'm the crazy one? I have been there and done that and I know the truth. I am the one in charge of these feelings.

This crazy-making has a name that I am all too familiar with. It has a name that brings me to again have to walk on egg shells. It has a name that makes me careful not to say too much or too little or the wrong thing. It has a name that makes me have to not be myself and to not be honest with what I know I see and feel. Again, I choose not to express it, and like a giant vacuum, I am being sucked back into a place I never wanted to return. It is my co-dependency that keeps me here and enables these feelings not to be addressed.

As long as I say nothing, then I am the one who enables these behaviors to continue.

Is it worth the journey back to become stronger so that I can again move beyond it? Maybe, if it is only a temporary stay, as my body, mind, spirit adjust to this new sense of well being.

Who is there to affirm this? Me? Who can listen and hear and comment back, and tell me, if this is really what is happening? Answers are only given when the questions are asked. There is never the presumption that a progress report is necessary. Maybe it is not necessary for others, but I just don't understand the process of healing that is taking place within me and I really want to know what is happening.

If I do not say what I am feeling then I am out of integrity. Something much bigger than I am guides me through the forces of my energy. It also blocks me and holds me back until the right moment happens. I pray that I know when to speak and when to be quiet. The words just flow out of me. I don't sit around planning what I should say.

My experience has taught me that I can trust my internal Spirit to guide me. I can "see" it all and probably have most of my life. If I resist these forces of energy, they come at me from another direction. I have said, "Lord make me an instrument of your peace" too many times and He heard me! I had to learn to trust and work with this very special intuitive gift.

I wrote the above, to help me let go of these thoughts rolling around in my head. This is about me and my issues of co-dependency. It was not to be for another six months before I would understand my preoccupation with these energies around me. These were connected to my sixth sense, as described by the author, Belleruth Naparstek in her book, *Your Sixth Sense: Activating Your Psychic Potential.* As a recovering co-dependent, I was used to having to rescue those around me in need. This process of healing for me was causing me to relive some of my past where secrets were guarded. These skeletons in the closet were much easier to ignore than to talk about them. It is these secrets and the "dance" created around them that bring about dysfunctional behaviors.

> **"The final wisdom of life requires not the annulment of incongruity, but the achievement of serenity within and above it."**
> **Reinhold Niebuhr**

Probably one of the greatest gifts that I was given in this whole process was the fact that during these very difficult moments, both physically and emotionally, I was not permitted to help anyone around me. I had to stay focused on my own healing. I took this very seriously at this point.

Some would ask why was this so important? It mattered to me only because it was part of my healing journey to know what I know, and to just "be" and not "be doing." To some people body language "speaks" loudly with unspoken words that never lie. I could hear what was not being said.

These signals reveal the things that the untrained "ear" may think go undetected. The effect on patient care and the doctor/patient relationships can be enormous when issues of control, structure and time lines are pushed to make people think an office is running properly. When patients cannot separate themselves from the energy that makes them uncomfortable, they stop coming in for their appointments, or change to another doctor, or therapist. If they are in school they find a different teacher. Some call it personality conflicts. I call it life!

This can be further explained with an experience I had in a dental office. For ten years that office was uncomfortable. My whole family knew. None of us ever wanted to be there. There was an energy force there that always felt so unhealthy, like an aura permeating throughout the entire office. Who the employees were, depended completely on what their boss thought they should or should not be. No one had an identity or dared to step out of line.

There were such controls in place that no one hardly spoke to anyone. They only did what they were told. As a family of seven, we all have very strong intuitions. We all tolerated this situation because it was in our dental plan to go to that particular dentist. Finally, when the children grew up, I went back to my former dentist and like a breath of fresh air, I felt such peace and contentment. Everyone was smiling! I felt so welcomed.

I remained in Chiropractic care because so many positive changes were happening to me and it really helped me stay accountable to a healthy life style I was enjoying. Biking became my exercise of choice and fifteen miles a day in the morning, several days a week was how I was doing it. It gave me the energy I needed to last until late at night! I was doing fine and I was never tired. What a difference all this had made to my life.

The Chiropractor loved his job and was good at the service he provided. It was good for me to have a safe quiet place where I could sort things out. I knew I had to focus my energies and my attention on my own healing. I could not "fix" those incongruities I saw in his staff that were calling out to me at that time. It was not my job and that was good!

CHAPTER THIRTEEN

The Mindbodyspirit Connection: Stepping Off The Roller Coaster

My healing journey wasn't over. When the student is ready, the teacher will appear! Those unexplained healers, helpers, wizards and guides continued to come into my life to help me explain me to myself! I was more than ready to learn. Nothing could stop me now, nor did I want it to.

Did I say, "I felt no empowerment?" I have thought about that often, since I first wrote it down three months ago. I guess I had to say it enough in order to release whatever was blocked within me and open the door to let the empowerment come through.

In my quest for knowledge I went to an International Conference on the Psychology of Health, Immunity and Disease. My energy was still out of control bouncing off the internal walls of my body. It had been eight weeks, since its release.

As an objective observer, subjectively feeling what I was observing, I was enjoying its effect on me. I was running each day in an effort to channel this added energy, as best I could. I wasn't talking much about the experience, but I sure could feel its effects and I liked it!

At the conference each morning for seven days I learned to center all this energy using a Kundalini form of Yoga taught by a wonderful teacher. She taught us how not only to focus my energy, but also how to release more of it, whenever we felt the need.

One technique, uses an energizing breath called the breath of fire. This is actually reversed breathing through your nose with your mouth closed. On the inhale your stomach will go out and on the exhale your abdomen moves in. Sitting in a chair you can do this any time and as rapidly as you feel you can move. Remember to keep your mouth closed so as not to hyperventilate! I have also used this successfully to clear my nasal passages when they get that "stuffed up" feeling. This works well for me!

I used a Yoga tape at first to learn the exercises. These exercises can be found in several different books on holistic health and alternative medicine. After that, I did them on my own throughout the day. I seldom feel tired any more at all. The back flexes I found to have great power. Also, focusing on correct posture has made a big difference to me.

Much of this was basic stretching exercises that I watched my children do before running track. The stretching can be done before even getting out of bed in the morning. These make getting up so much easier. Create your own early morning routine before your feet even hit the floor. Keep them simple and then add new ones as you feel comfortable. Do it informally without any guilt!

My daughter encouraged me to do some sit ups. She calls them "crunches". I was so proud to be able to do one and then two each morning before I got out of bed. She went off to Germany for two months to study. When she came back I was doing five a day! She does five hundred! She told me that was great. Now several months later I am doing forty a day each morning.

Make the exercises fun and laugh at yourself while you push yourself through any internal resistance that might want to tell you, "You can't". The accomplishment will make such a difference to you.

I started out the same way on my bicycle. I was so proud of doing three miles of biking a day four days a week. I didn't rush. I just added a mile here and there and picked a favorite time of day to go out. Now I bike fifteen miles a day, five days a week and I love it. I go out early in the morning so that the energy stays with me all day.

Energy is not anything I am having difficulty finding these days. Doing any kind of exercise is a good way to clear your head while you have conversations with your Spirit Guide. Sometimes you even cross paths with a neighbor. Just keep things simple and keep smiling.

Getting up in the morning is so much easier for me now. My legs actually support me and I feel more like starting my day. I was so off balance before I began Chiropractic care. This gave me something to believe in and helped me make myself accountable to me!

You need only to begin. Find something you want to do. Believe in it and listen to your body. I found these very pleasant and not difficult, as long as I listened to my body.

On the very first morning of the conference, during my first lesson in Yoga, I noticed that while sitting on the floor in a comfortable, relaxed position my chin centered off to the right about seven degrees. This didn't bother me, but I did notice it two or three times in the first hour and a half.

That morning I began a three day pre-conference program for a Mindbody Medicine Certification involving several facilitators. I found myself very conscious of my discomfort in the chair. I wanted to sit up straight, but was having difficulty. The presenter was off was off my right shoulder. I found myself moving often to stay comfortable and square - for lack of another word.

To say that co-dependency has been a major issue for me would be a bit of an understatement. These past few months I have worked so hard to let go of it. This has been such an integral part of my healing journey, since I know the stress it produces in my life affects my neck.

Anyhow, that morning, along with giving us wonderful information, the workshop facilitator had us do an exercise in guided imagery. This process uses visualization to create mental movies with positive images of health and wholeness that help to relax the body. These reprogram the mind to promote healing and bring peace and harmony within.

We closed our eyes and I was asked to picture an issue that was presently a part of my life. We were to visualize it — move it out away from us, play with it for a moment and then let it go…. So…this is what happened to me in the process:

> I pictured myself face down on the adjustment table in the chiropractor's office surrounded by my sense of entrapment inside this psychological cloud of co-dependency. It hung directly above me for a while where it stayed "looking" at me.

> I was then told to move it away. What I did was not sweep it out the door, but rather, using the word "sucked in" in reverse I let this cloud get "sucked out" the door and down the hall. In my mind's eye it then hesitated a moment, turned, and pulled with it my extended cloud of co-dependency surrounding the chiropractic assistant in my doctor's office. She was my co-dependent whom had been trying to rescue from burnout, and then subsequently detach from in the process of refocusing on my own issues.

With both clouds now together, they continued being sucked down the hall and out the front door. I quickly closed the door, feeling safe inside, slamming it shut, happy to be free of its entrapment. The facilitator gently continued, "Now play with it for a while!" I didn't want to play with this cloud of co-dependency. I wanted it out of my life - forever! But I did what I was told!

In my mind, again, I reluctantly went outside the front door and dragged this cloud of entrapment across the parking lot and pushed it into the ditch by the road. I then shoved it under the driveway out of sight. I buried it forever. At that moment I felt a complete release and inner peace.

When we were finished, several people shared what they had experienced. Some had gone to sleep. The facilitator asked if anyone had found closure on an issue. I described what had just happened indicating previously, my great discomfort in having to be a patient in need, and also, my life long journey to free myself of my co-dependency issues. I told the group that the guided imagery had been successful because I had been working really hard these past few months on letting go and lightening up.

When we broke for lunch, my table partner, a medical physician, asked my permission to comment on what she saw in me and ask if she could ask me some questions. The first thing she said was "Congratulations." I thought, "For what?" Was it for what I said or did? I knew something had happened, but such a strong word. It should have happened. It was the logical consequence of my process. I was so ready to really let go of the control this issue had over me.

She also asked me, if I perceived energy? I said "Yes, I can feel energy, but I cannot see it." She then said, "You will be pleased. If you're not comfortable with this then please tell me." I told her, "I'm fine, thank you. You may go on."

She continued. "You are not the same person you were when we met this morning. You are very changed. I do not know the center of your injury or illness, but after you sat down from sharing your experience, I saw all the energy release itself around your neck and your color return to your body." I listened, knowing exactly what she was saying. "I sensed also that you are not comfortable with your role as a patient."

How true! I told her of my challenge to concentrate on my own healing and to not be concerned with the issues of those around me who perhaps in my judgment also needed some healing. There was also an incongruity in my role, as a patient in relationship to my doctor. She so wisely suggested that this too needs be healed in order for me to heal. This was to happen in its own time, as I let go of any unwillingness I might have to trust my own intuitive knowledge. I was getting there.

This experience with guided imagery that morning definitely took me off the "roller coaster" that for years had given me emotional highs and lows. Almost immediately, I noticed this. My husband affirmed this a month later. He thought it was wonderful and definitely a difference. This freedom was long overdue. Over Christmas I taught him Yoga which we did together for two weeks while on vacation. This had a healing affect on him also. What fun! We really needed to add more fun to our lives. These past few years had been tough on both of us.

I always admired those who could remain emotionally constant in all situations. It's tough to become that way when you have been conditioned, since childhood, to "hop to it," and then to have to walk on egg shells most of your life fearful of when the next crisis would occur that you thought you had to fix!!

Something else happened earlier that day, as if there could be more! There had been another guided imagery, a simple one, where we were asked to bring ourselves to a place of happiness and peacefulness.

I imagined myself running on the beach. I felt burdened and heavy, not a lot, but definitely sensed a resistance, as I ran. This actually had happened the night before in real life.

I love to run, but looking at my life from the inside out, I was always running up hill. I now know that this had a lot to do with my neck injury from long ago and the emotional burdens I carried on my shoulders all these years.

As I continued to run in my mind, I pictured myself dropping the burdens of my life on the beach, as if they were a heavy jacket or sweatshirt. Finally, I was running like a free spirit. No longer did I feel any resistance.

I was free, winning the race, saying, "Yes!" and clinching my hand, as if to lock in the experience into my memory, as a trigger for later reference. I, actually, felt the power of the experience within me.

What was interesting about all this was that three days later the temperature reached seventy. I went out on the beach and began to run. The difference between Monday and Wednesday was awesome. All that I had pictured in my guided imagery transpired. It was sunset with the full moon rising at the same time. I could have run for miles watching the moonlight dance on top of the ocean waves.

This conference became a personal retreat. I created the following guidelines for me to follow during that week:

- No music/radio/television
- Eat lightly with food I prepared
- Pay attention to me and listened to my body
- Keep silent and to myself
- Answer in class only when it felt right
- Remain non-judgmental of the views of others
- Walk or ran on the beach each day
- Take time to watch the sun set and moon rise
- Attend Yoga class each day and practice
- Set goals for continued exercise and other healthy habits

Belleruth Naparstek, a practicing psychotherapist, is the author of *Staying Well with Guided Imagery* and creator of the Health Journeys series of guided imagery audiotapes. She explains that "Guided imagery takes us beyond clock time into a different type of time. It transcends the limits with our mind and creates an altered state that makes us more ready to rewrite the script of our life that immobilizes us and inhibits personal growth." Every time a trigger sparks the memory of a traumatic event, she suggests that we change the script. An example would be to remember the success I felt running freely on the beach.

Another quiet affirmation might be to picture and experience the feeling the love of everyone who has ever loved you in your lifetime or the kindness of a special person who has been your healer, helper, wizard or guide.

When the feelings connected to a particular trauma overwhelm you, step outside of them. Talk about them, as if they were a movie. Rewrite the story breaking it down into smaller bites to diffuse the emotional charge.

When my feelings of entrapment were getting to me and

releasing my own issues of abuse, I had to shift my focus to the positive outcomes of my good health that I was already experiencing. Only then could I realize and accept that it was not the intention of anyone around me to hurt me. I could choose to accept their love which I have always known was buried in their anger.

I had to separate the two issues and not let the two feelings run together. I had to practice this for quite a while. When I would feel anxious and vulnerable, I would use the imagery described earlier in Chapter Ten to reclaim my strength. This allowed me to detach from the pain and avoid getting drawn into the drama. By inserting the image of a person from whom I have received unconditional love, such as my father, into the place where the image of the person who hooks me resides, I can objectively see the nature of the hook, as it changes my consciousness.

Imagery helps me to see my choices to engage or disengage from the hook. I stay focused and respond from a centered mode paying close attention to the response of my body. It becomes a form of receptive imagery where I choose to respond out of love and not resistance.

Remaining conscious of my breathing, I am able to go inside and rest peacefully. Our breath is a way into the soul. This quiet process reminded me that wounds heal from the inside out. Some of these wounds are deep and may require more time to heal.

I am grateful to have a safe place where I could think this through and let go of it. I try to pay attention to my need for this silence often now during the course of the day. It helps me to focus and gives me a moment of quiet meditation. It has made such a difference in the way I feel and in the way I project myself.

So much of our pain is locked up in the somatic or body cells. Guided imagery puts that pain beyond the wall so that we can accelerate the healing process, as we identify with the best powerful image for change.

The temptation is to hold on to the pain. It has been a part of my essence for so long. Who will I be without it? What will fill the void when it is gone? A part of me does not want to give up the memory that serves to protect me. The memory has become the teacher. However letting go of the teacher and keeping the lesson permits me to stay sensitive to the needs of others in similar situations - something that is important to me. I must also mourn the loss of who I was in my pain and celebrate who I have become in my freedom.

"With insights come change."
                                          Milton Erickson

My dear friend, Judy Webster, asked me, "What color do you see now that all those tough feelings have moved on? What did you replace them with?" My answer to her was simply, "The color of calm."

I was enjoying every minute of it! Since that time, now a year later, my emotional roller coaster has never returned and the "color of calm" is beautiful!

CHAPTER FOURTEEN

Emerging Wisdom As Life
Changes To A New Direction

Returning home to Michigan after my week of mindbodyspirit renewal my doctor asked me what went on for me while I was there? He had a unique way of sensing my energy fields. There had been an enormous number of positive changes.

I wasn't sure how much I wanted to tell him. To me most of it was pretty profound. In fact I asked his permission first on a few accounts. I felt that it was time for me to move on, but I had become a patient patient. I really wanted the rest of the story and still believed he knew something I wanted to know.

I reflected on a very interesting experience from Bernie Siegel's post-conference workshop. He is a medical doctor who does a lot of work reading the self-portraits of many of his cancer patients and helping them find their areas of emotional resistance.

As participants, Dr. Siegel had us draw a picture of ourselves in our present situation. Having so successfully completed that guided imagery six days earlier, which literally took me off my emotional roller coaster of a lifetime, I decided to just draw a picture of me face down on the adjustment table in the office of the Chiropractor. It sort of felt like that was where I had been living these days and the drawing was no big deal to me. I was feeling a little brain dead on overload from the intensity of the week, but I did the drawing anyhow.

My self-portrait that day was as follows:

Simply drawn, the doctor was standing at my feet, tall and separate, with his activator tool in his hand. Everything was in black and white except for me. I was dressed in bright colors, dressed in purple and blue with my brown hair. The doctor looked like an ethereal figure, very tall and distant, almost like a shadow standing at my feet.

While the rest of the group finished their drawings, I took a break, and left the room for a minute. When I returned, groups had formed to discuss their drawings with a partner. Bernie was overseeing the activity, but was not connected to any one group, so I asked him, if he would review my drawing. I told him about my experience with the guided imagery earlier in the week and its impact on me. I also told him briefly about my issues of co-dependency connected with my experiences in Chiropractic care.

With one quick look the interpretation of my picture was obvious.

Even with my face hidden in the table, my body was alive and vibrant wearing the colors of purple, blue and brown which reflect good health, spirituality and tranquility. The vanishing effect of the doctor's portrait indicated the character of a true healer.

Having facilitated the natural processes of my healing with his healing energy, my drawing showed that it was now his time to release me and set me free, so that I could become in the true sense, a healer to others. In the drawing the Chiropractor looked lifeless and now ineffective, perhaps indicating that it was my time to move on. His job was complete.

"Ask to be released," was suggested to me. "Your drawing indicates that he is through with you and that you no longer need him. The true healer, or shaman, accomplishes his or her task and then releases the patient, so that he or she can focus their healing energy on someone else."

"This completion sets the patient free, as in your case, to be a healer to others." This is to me a true definition of healer - an angel placed in my life, as my teacher and guide to help me move to the next level of understanding the path of my life's journey. There is a time for coming and a time for letting go. "Perhaps, even now you are to be set free to become his healer helping him to understand the power and influence of the co-dependency issues in his life."

Bernie noticed that the cloud of co-dependency over me was gone from my drawing. My doctor had been my spiritual healer in mindbodyspirit. He was the person to whom I silently made myself accountable for every goal I set. He, like many other healers, helpers, wizards and guides who have touched my life knew nothing about this. He facilitated the natural process of healing within me.

The doctor did not have to know what I did to make it happen. That part was for me. My mindbodyspirit did the rest of the work.

I was feeling so free! For years I had helped others understand how their issues of self-esteem were connected to their issues of co-dependency. I loved being part of their empowerment. As a story teller using my own unique signature stories, I gave people permission to share their stories and consequently bring the support of others to them. This united all of us in the universality of our feelings. Did this new found freedom mean I could now get back to doing what I truly believed to be my purpose and mission in life? Time would only tell.

I felt excitement and peace. I was so grateful for all the opportunities these past six months had brought to me. I was also thankful that I had been the recipient of my doctor's care. I also thanked myself for taking the time to trust the healing process and participate in the journey.

Back at the chiropractor's office on my next visit, after sharing my story, I again became a very patient patient. I did not know what this all meant to him, but I sure knew what it meant to me. My appointment schedule did not change.

The energy around the office still made me feel very uncomfortable, but I remained present and chose to stay detached, riding on the wonderful glow I felt from my conference and retreat. I also had just spent two weeks in Florida over Christmas with my husband. Here in Michigan, winter was upon us, again, but my attitude had changed entirely from the year before.

Exercising regularly was probably one of the most important factors governing the way I was feeling. I had kept up my walking and running schedule which I began in the summer, and continued to do some biking.

I also began to notice a big change in the way my husband was feeling. He was really doing very well, so we were again a healthy team. I know he had been worried about me for a long time, even though he did not say anything until after the fact.

I chose to continue in Chiropractic care and stayed focused, getting centered and quiet and praying for whatever was to be during each visit. I tried not to think about the unanswered questions that still roamed through my head, although many of them had been answered.

The conference had really helped me with the cognitive piece, introducing me to current authors on the topics of my experiences and giving me a chance to reconnect with my biology, psychology and philosophy background. My empowerment came, as a result of the stimulation created by all these magnificent "teachers." To have spent the week with so many like-minds was so enriching.

Many, many people have helped me to understand the changes that I experienced along this journey. They have all been so honest. Understanding the biological mechanisms of the brain and its power to affect change in our body, were very powerful lessons for me.

I was a true participant in the learning process. Each day unfolded revealing new insights to me. I was so ready to listen and I was feeling so free-spirited throughout my day. I knew I was now healing rapidly.

The people who attended the conference genuinely shared their hope for an integration of many healing modalities. From this will come a new kind of medicine that involves a partnership where teaching is as important as the treatment, and personal responsibility for self-care is empowered through self-awareness, relaxation, meditation, nutrition and exercise.

James S. Gordon, M.D., expresses this in his book, *Manifesto for a New Medicine.* "The new medicine fosters an optimistic and hopeful attitude toward the experience of illness. It is based on a therapeutic relationship that is more egalitarian than authoritative. It creates a new synthesis of ancient and modern, conventional and unconventional techniques, the best of modern science and the most enduring aspects of perennial medical wisdom."

I was feeling so much better. One day at a time over the past seven months, I was getting my strength back in my legs and in my hands. I was feeling more balance and my new found energy was a wonderful treat. The Yoga and exercise had really helped me keep all this energy focused.

Friends who had not seen me for a while, would ask me with great intent, "What was going on? What was I doing?" They wanted some of what I had! It was that obvious because I had a real positive energy about me that I could feel. My friends were actually telling me that I had a glow about me. There was an internal glow there too!

These changes are in me, facilitated by the "healing process" that was taking place within me. My weight has not changed, but my physical body has changed greatly. Yes, this can be overwhelming, if I let it be and if I really want to explore the impact on me psychologically and spiritually. But I chose to enjoy the present moments with these good feelings and do some more exploring later.

During my appointment time I kept up my same procedure. My visits were now twice a week instead of three times a week. I felt my S-shaped neck curve had changed and I really wanted to see it. I figured that besides everything else that had happened in the last eight months, my neck was still my primary concern. No one had told me that it should be otherwise.

Friends, my healers, helpers, wizards and guides closest to me, were asking me again why I continued in this doctor's care when I truly believed my neck was cured and I physically was feeling so good? Surprise of surprise! This was fast becoming a "never ending story."

We looked at the X-ray of my neck. It had changed in the right direction, but it was not yet perfect. Remember, the doctor said, he could fix it. What I was experiencing was the difference between being healed and cured. I was feeling very healed, but I was not cured yet!

Janet Quinn, Ph.D., defines healing as, "the emergence of right relationship at or among any one or more levels of the human experience. Curing is the elimination of the signs and symptoms of disease."

She explains that "healing may occur without curing and that curing may also occur without healing. Curing may not always be possible, yet healing is always possible. Curing is predictable while healing is always creative and unpredictable in both process and outcome."

After looking at my X-ray I quietly told my doctor, "My neck did not straighten out completely, but my heart and soul and spirit did. You again teach me humility and patience."

Remember I said, I was going to be the perfect patient because I was always the perfect child growing up! Isn't it amazing how quickly we can fall into the comfortable roles we played in our family systems. And so! The journey continues.

I was disappointed, but chose to continue. For two months I was riding on the good energy I was feeling and my peacefulness that I had found within. I could not figure out why I was unable to stop analyzing everything around me. My Spirit Guide was working overtime and never minded a minute of it. I knew part of it was my commitment to continue Chiropractic care.

This whole process was wearing me down and I wanted to get on with my life in my time and not God's time, even though I knew everything happens in its own time! I knew I had to trust God's time and let go again.

This was very difficult for me. No matter how hard I tried I could not shut off whatever was out there affecting me. I knew this discomfort could be explained through the eyes of my recovering co-dependency and asked for an extended time to talk about it. I could not go where I was not invited, yet I sensed that there was a real interest on the part of my doctor in finding some explanation for my confusion. Finally, I took the courage to ask for this consultation.

I explained what I was feeling in reference to what I thought was a lack of choices and options in my care. We come, complete our task and leave. I did not like feeling as if I were a "number." I felt privileged to be in his care. I also believe that as a patient, I have given him the privilege to work with me, not just on me. It is the healing touch connected to the heart that helps the body heal.

This is all forgotten when healers get into a "got-to-get-the-job-done mode." It transforms their healing hands into procedural hands looking for information. They may see many patients, but for what purpose, if the process of healing slows down because they remain disconnected. Patients know this insensitive behavior is working against their desire to heal. When a person is injured and in pain he or she becomes vulnerable. When feelings are shut out something very special within each of us is lost. It is that part of us which makes us human and not just a machine!

> **Throughout this process, I was greatly affected by what I call communication deprivation. This occurs when patients feel so rushed that they do not have the courage to interrupt the timing and ask the questions they have in their heart.**

The gift of time is an opportunity for reflection, or prayer, in our lives directed towards the common good of all. Each visit while I waited, I used my time alone for that purpose. It served as the foundation for my faith and trust and carried me through many personal challenges.

I came to accept the fact that the time any doctor gives to his or her patients is all the time he or she can allow. In some ways this is a form of control, as it becomes a condition that restricts unconditional love and the natural flow within the learning process.

My nature is such that it is so easy for me to compromise my own needs so that other patients wouldn't have to wait longer. For several chapters now I have talked about escaping from those things that rob me of my peacefulness. Here I was again in the middle of them.

I was learning so much. I figured there still had to be a reason for all this. I certainly knew it was good for me to be there. My husband encouraged me to stay with it. He knew the positive and healthy effects all this had on me. He also knew I was no longer on the emotional roller coaster and that felt good. Emotions and feelings are what make us human, but the emotional roller coaster makes us tough to live with! Who me?

The mobility in my neck was as excellent as it was when I was a child. I felt energetic enough and was seldom tired.

I was getting very interesting "power surges" in the night in the form of hot flashes. They were always comfortable and gave me a true sense of peacefulness and a quiet chuckle. I never minded them. If they woke me up, I didn't fight them. I embraced the energy and if I could not roll back to sleep, I got up, took care of some things and went back to bed when I felt tired.

Keeping up my goals for exercise and eating properly made such a difference in my life. They had become part of my inner fiber. None was considered "work" anymore. My muscles had also become quite firm so that I no longer felt like I was in training.

The physical appearance and the shape of my body had changed. I was drinking a lot of water. I was still biking and doing stretches and Yoga in the morning, very informally, but still doing them. I also got the strength back in my right hand and I was staying healthy with no prescription drugs throughout the winter months.

My curly hair came back after twenty-eight years. I also had lost all my cravings for chocolate and sweets and could no longer tolerate much beef. I ate nothing with aspartame in it and watched my intake of "fatty foods".

It had definitely been a good choice to stay in chiropractic care these months and walk through the "storm." I had such clarity of thought. I really had wanted that back for a long time.

My relationship with my husband was also very good, especially since we have chosen to respond out of love and not resistance. I practiced only seeing the good in people. Long ago I had stopped listening to any negatives thoughts connected to broken promises.

The chiropractic assistant took a new job in a different place. She was my support person and I missed her. Through all those weeks of turmoil, she had made it safe for me. When things got crazy, she always affirmed my feelings. I didn't want to change anyone around me. I only needed to change me and at that point in time that was a full time job.

When I felt I wasn't being listened to, she shared her story of healing and confusion and helped me understand that my feelings were, perhaps, also part of my process. She always directed my questions back to the doctor with such respect. She served as a sounding board for my feelings of incompleteness and unresolved issues. We shared our understanding of co-dependency issues and saw our need to set boundaries and limits for ourselves in the times of confusion and insecurity.

When we become dependent on others to fulfill our needs, we also may get angry at them when they can no longer fulfill those needs. It is our expectation that get in the way. This just becomes another lesson in letting go.

If we put a lot of anger into our body, then our body will want more food, drink, chocolate and other things to fill all that emptiness and make us feel better. But sadly, we don't feel better.

Forgiveness is one way out of all these unfulfilled expectations. Letting go of unresolved conflicts, or the misbehavior of others, is another. My whipped-lashed neck was an old injury; my co-dependency was also an old injury; I wasn't born with them. They grew out things that happened to me along the way. Letting go of the pain they caused in my life and accepting that which is, exactly as it is, renews my spirit and gives me back my faith in me and my God who created me as I am.

My Spirit Guide and wonderful internal counselor brought out many healing emotions in me over these past months, but anger wasn't one of them. At least not as an anger directed at anyone. Maybe this was because I had already done that chapter in my life! My anger now translated itself into a sadness.

The process of change often requires the process of grieving, as we acknowledge those things in our lives which, at first, we denied and now fully understand. We are able to incorporate these new lessons into the very essence of who we have become and let go of the discomfort and pain they previously caused in our lives.

The sense of being controlled without choices was very strong inside of me. I was unable to let go of my expectation that things should be different from what they were. These feelings were trying to tell me to trust God's time in finding out the answers to my questions, or for others to change and grow.

I was again feeling trapped. I had forgotten that the healing of these issues is a process and sometimes when we have not quite learned the lesson, these issues will resurface just to test us again until we really learn them and can move beyond them.

I had tried detachment. Separation was another choice. This was a strange perception of an office where the intention was to project the complete opposite of this - a sense of peacefulness and safety. Or were all these feelings just inside of me?

CHAPTER FIFTEEN

Healthy Detachment:
The Power Of Choice

I finally decided it was time for me to take a break, a real break. The doctor immediately knew I was up to something and asked me what was going on. He could always sense a change in my energy patterns. "Today is my last appointment," I told him. I had to get out of there. I had tried so hard to detach. After ten months, enough was enough for me, even though I knew that, unless I resolved the issues that were holding me there, they were going to follow me everywhere I went.

We talked for a while. The doctor again explained the process to me and why it was important that I stay and continue in Chiropractic care. I was very sad and felt defeated. I felt we were both learning the same lessons, as reflections of one another. Although so many things had changed in my life and all for the better, I was not able to completely block out certain energies. Separation from them would allow me to clear my own head. I did not make that decision when we finished talking, nor did I make my next appointment.

Dr. John DeMartini in his book, *Count Your Blessings, The Healing Power of Gratitude and Love*, says that whatever you run away from, you run into...We can't escape our fears because they stem from within us... We continue to attract lessons until we learn their messages, appreciate

**their blessings, and bring the dualism of our
lopsided perceptions into perfect balance."**

Knowing I could change no one, I felt I had to protect
myself from me! I only could change me and my reaction to
others. I just wanted some time to step back and try to objectively understand what I was feeling. So much had happened
and it was all new and good. In some ways leaving would
have been like quitting weight watchers when everything
was going along as scheduled. What was I doing and why?

So I had this dream to help me understand. This was
only the second one in the year that I remembered, since I
entered Chiropractic care.

The Dream

It was 5:04 AM, as the alarm went off. "I was being
chased to the edge of a cliff by someone large, not
frightening, just someone large with power over
me. I had to make a decision. I had to decide to
either be captured or to jump. There was a big city
below and the rocky cliff was very steep and went
straight down. There was someone running with
me, but more as a shadow, than a specific person.

As I went to jump, I slipped, my hands remaining
on the edge of the cliff. This being caught me.
Reaching down it took my hand to help me. It could
fly like superman. I sensed it was not really after
me. I felt safe, but not totally out of danger because
we were both dropping very quickly a long distance
to the ground. This being was having fun going so
fast that I sternly asked it to please slow down, or I
would be hurt when we landed.

Since this being was holding on to me, as we
dropped, I felt gratitude for its saving me, so I
hugged and thanked this being for helping me.

As I looked at it, the being had turned into a rubber mannequin and could not respond. I woke up. I assumed I landed safely. I was not frightened."

The significance of this to me reflected my desire to escape the confines that I chose to participate in through Chiropractic care. There were two forces working inside of me: one that wanted to stay because it was good for me to be there and one that wanted to leave because a part of me believed that I could not heal any further within these circumstances. I felt obligated and trapped, unable to say to anyone who would understand, what was holding me back.

With the gift of non-judgment often comes the practice of non-response. Add to that the limitations bestowed upon us by time and you have peace at all costs.

I was looking into this nonperson for something to identify with on a personal level, perhaps the sharing of a story. I genuinely felt that this lack of verbal response, placed all the burden of understanding on me and forced me to go within for my answers. Of course, if that hadn't happened, then I wouldn't have met my Spirit Guide and by now we had become inseparable friends. What didn't I understand?

I read every piece of information in the office and it was good information, but what was happening to me was not written there. I went on the internet. It wasn't there either. I again felt very raw and dismantled. Little did I know that I was actually being given everything that I needed at the time. I was fully empowered and had become my own healer paying full attention to my mind, body and spirit, but in that moment I could not make that connection.

Dan Millman in his book, *Laws of Spirit* suggests that "It is only when you reclaim the power to end a relationship that you can fully commit to it.

**It becomes your choice to stay, and you stay, not
because you have to, but because you want to.
That is when your life changes from an obligation
to a blessed opportunity. That's when miracles
happen!"**

When I left the doctor's office that day everything in my
body fell apart, as if I had never gone for any care all these
past ten months. I knew differently, but my body did not
know. Every ounce of stress I felt centered itself in my neck,
shoulders and back. I raised my monitor on my computer; I
changed my chair; nothing could make me comfortable.

It was a long thirty-six hours before I made the decision
again to continue in this doctor's care. I was not going to give
up Chiropractic care. I had experienced its power and truly
believe in its philosophy. I was just not going to continue in
this doctor's care and not for any reason in his awareness. My
reasons were my own, connected to my need to separate
myself from the things I could not change. These were my
issues of co-dependency to a system that pulled me in. I
wanted what it could give me, but I no longer wanted the
roller coaster ride I had stepped down from three months
ago.

Finally, acknowledging my pain I told myself that I
could make an appointment and go back the next day, if I
needed to. After that I would find another doctor when I did
not hurt as much. Immediately, with that decision every
muscle in my body relaxed. It was like a wave of motion
passing through me.

Our thoughts can give such power to our mind! Nothing
hurt anymore. In fact I did not go in the next day, but waited
until the following week. The pain all stayed away and was
replaced with enough energy that I cleaned my attic and
organized my basement that weekend while my husband
went skiing!

Detachment would have allowed me to stay there, as an objective observer. I had tried that for ten months, but it did not work well for me. I remained too subjective, even though I had improved.

Because of the more than five hundred seminars and workshops I have presented on the topic of co-dependency and self-esteem over the past twelve years, I understand, so clearly, the complexity and influence these issues have on our lives. I walked my talk and now through this journey, I've walked it again, but with a much deeper involvement. I never thought any of this would happen again! To stay in this doctor's care was a significant part of my healing journey towards wholeness in mindbodyspirit. I certainly had not yet arrived at inner peace.

Within a co-dependent system, everyone becomes a participant, much like a family member who works hard to maintain identity within the family system. In a healthy environment, reality is truthful. Individuals are allowed to be themselves, as they are, independent of one another.

In a co-dependent environment people easily lose their identity and their reality, as they must follow the rules of those who are in charge of them, or control them. Everyone is affected. They cover for one another and they start to become what they are expected to be and not who they truly are. Their individuality is lost along with their self-esteem. People get quiet; they get angry and they hold that anger inside because they will be judged, criticized and blamed if they open up or do anything creative or out of line. Sometimes guidelines are not clear, yet in a controlled environment, the expectation is that they know the rules anyway.

This is why certain health professionals have difficulty keeping their office staff and even some of their patients or clients. If these patients have detachment skills, they can stay.

If they do not, then for their own peace of mind, they will choose to separate themselves from the environment that makes them uncomfortable.

Those who leave have had enough control in their life and do not want to be controlled by anyone or anything anymore! Today's young people are particularly vulnerable to this because they have been taught the power of choice. If they find they cannot be themselves, or that their talents are being wasted, they will choose another practitioner or another job.

Unfortunately, they may also choose another spouse for the same reason. The little picture becomes the big picture and they feel trapped and unable to see their choice to change their attitude towards their situation. Working it through may not be an option for them because of their determination to be in charge of their own happiness.

Isn't that intuitive? And I learned that all in silence! This was the basis for so many of my difficulties, as a patient. I knew I could have explained this system to whoever might want to listen, but nobody asked me! There was no reason to ask.

What is normal is normal and who is to say that it isn't? So I let it go and detached and detached again. Within the allotted time of an appointment this could not be discussed because the issue for me was so deep, but I did have to at least resolve it in my mind before I could truly be healed.

For two years prior to my neck injury, as a visitor, I sat in occasionally on my husband's and son's chiropractic adjustments with my same doctor. I never felt any of these issues in their presence with him, but then I was not the patient. In fact I thought I was a friend. When I became a patient, then somehow instantaneously there were a new set of rules.

I did not like that. I know now that this was part of my incongruity of role I felt as a patient. I needed to address it as my own issue because it certainly was not an issue for the doctor.

All I wanted was to be the doctor's friend, get better and move on, but I had to first be a patient his way. Blindly, I chose to do that. I will not judge any of this as right or wrong. These were my feeling and no one ever told me they were wrong. In fact I always felt safe enough to think for myself because I was never judged. This was very important to me.

I trusted him as my doctor. His presence was very kind. With each visit I was physically feeling so much stronger and balanced. Emotionally, I was really working at letting go and spiritually, I was learning to trust my God!

I continued in his care. I tried so hard not to not let these things affect me. So often though, I felt like I was left out there to fend for myself, but if I did not push the system and speak my truth, then this was my problem. When I did get up enough courage to address the issues with him, he was always very receptive and listened to me. These conversations always left me peaceful and with some closure, but they never quite explained the depth of my experience.

Once I could say what was going on for me and recognized from where these feelings originated, the controls over me lost their power and they were no longer begging my attention.

This was about nine months after I began in Chiropractic care. I relaxed and continued to enjoy a more peaceful journey over the next few months. In retrospect I was very glad that I had decided to stay and continue in his care.

Writing this book has clarified these feelings for me as I take full ownership of these experiences as part of my journey to wholeness. These are powerful lessons. I cannot blame anyone else for my feelings. If others do not understand my issues then I cannot expect them to be able to take me any further in understanding them then they are willing to go themselves as they are a reflection of me. These are powerful lessons for me.

"Responding with love and not resistance" I have done this with my church; I have done it with my children and my husband, why not now with my doctor? I have let go of any expectation I might have had, that he should be anyone, but who he is. He is a good person and he does his job well. He loves what he does. No one has the right to rob him of that joy. I have learned so much from him in his silence and who am I to judge what might be right or wrong for anyone else? He does what he does and he does it well. I never doubted that, or lost my trust in his abilities as a Chiropractor.

My Spirit Guide was right there with me through all of this, as I continued to listen in silence. My questions began to subside, one by one, as I let go of the words in my head and arrived at a place where true healing could occur.

The simple decision, to choose to continue in a program that was definitely good for me, gave me back my sense of freedom and choice. I became more honest and trusted that it was all right to be me - to think, as I think, and to be who I am.

This has truly been a journey back to self! If I did not take this journey, then I would not be able to help others move beyond that place in my journey that I would not go myself. I cannot give to others what I do not have for myself. It takes courage to see this and to understand its power.

"Remember Who You Are," the sign read, as I entered the Church of St. Francis Assisi in New York City the following weekend. I remembered!

CHAPTER SIXTEEN

Responding Out of Love
And Not Resistance

Good things were happening. There was a lot of healing going on in many places in my life and the only thing I thought I needed to heal was a crooked neck from my sailing injury many months ago. I could not deny my miracles. It had been four years since my parents died and I broke my leg. Three years had passed since our last two children of five moved out of our house and went off to college. For the first time in thirty years we did not have to go anywhere or be anywhere with our children. They were all off on their own and doing well.

Along this journey back to self, I chose to use this time wisely to rebuild our marriage of thirty years which for obvious reasons needed to be redirected back on us, as a couple, and not as a family of seven. This became an absolute priority in both of our lives and I would let go of everything material in order to do it.

My husband was my college buddy. Together we shared many dreams for the past thirty years. Why not take it through another thirty or forty, as did our parents?

We were best friends for two years before we even dated. We danced and sang together in college. We have always loved music. He was from Washington, D.C. I was from New York. When I was eighteen and he was nineteen, he was one of the first students I met on Wheeling College campus five hundred miles from home.

We dated four years on through graduate school in the days when couples didn't sleep together before they got married. We shared dreams and even named our first two children, as my Mom would say, "Long before they were even a twinkle in God's eye!"

We were in school together the day Kennedy was shot. He was in an accounting class; I was standing outside in the hall waiting to tell him what had happened. John F. Kennedy was "our" President!

We got married for all the right reasons and even promised one another we didn't want to do the things our parents, our wonderful parents, did that we did not like! But there we were. Ten years into our marriage, we had become just like them doing all those things to our children, which we did not like done to us, as kids growing up. Two months after we were married my husband's parents had sent us an article entitled, "Like Father Like Son!" I still have that article. Did they know something we didn't know? It crept up on us when we weren't looking. Those particular parts of our personalities did not get along, and created a rough ten years for both of us, when the children were young.

Like many, who were products of the fifties and sixties, we never ever thought our lives or the lives of our children would be so influenced by the experiences of our past. As Robert Subby writes in his book, *Lost in the Shuffle: The Co-dependent Reality*, we were raised with many dysfunctional rules. These were carried over from the olden days and worked during that place in time, but they did not apply today or even make sense anymore.

As healers, helpers, wizards and guides to others, it became our job to sort out those rules and separate the good ones from the not so good. This created many conflicts that confused the two of us greatly. We had to learn what should be kept and what could be thrown away. Those stories are what led me to write the book, *Does Anyone Hear Our Cries for Help?* We were crying out for help while not understanding the incongruities of love and hate in our lives and in the world around us.

> **Together we had more invested on the good side of things with our home, our family and friends, our Church and our children, than could ever be weighed down by the mountains of stuff we have had to climb through in order to see ourselves clear.**

Our life together was a thirty year investment in my mind, body, and spirit that had created who we are today. We never wanted to let go of one another otherwise I'm sure we would have. Often there were times while we were in our confusion that we could not even communicate. Instead we held on tight in silence, knowing that the depth of our connection was far beyond the pain we were feeling.

We never wanted to hurt one another, but at times we did. There was so much craziness that we could not understand. We didn't even know how we got to this point. We were just there.

> **We were very different from one another, yet deep down where it really counted, we were very much the same.**

Our commitment to our marriage was a covenant and a very strong value for us. It was a promise to one another and we wanted to keep that promise. Although at times, that thought didn't even seem to enter the picture. The root of that belief was always there, buried somewhere. Hurting people hurt people and when you're hurting it's difficult to see beyond the present moment.

We had to learn to ask for the support we needed from each other in order to handle the tough issues. No one has to do this alone but, also understand that no one will help, unless we ask. In those days that was something I never knew how to do that very well. I feared the judgment of others and kept my secrets. We both did.

We now realize how much time we both wasted blaming one another for our unhappiness and thinking we could change the other person. Why we ever thought we had that right is beyond me. Personalities are what personalities are. We have been together all these years because it was in our differences that we found the compliment of who we were for one another. We have now established our individuality and addressed our co-dependency issues. We have come to accept these differences that now seemed less important with the children no longer living at home.

Our present relationship centers around our responding out of love and not out of resistance. The things in our lives that are most difficult for us to accept in one another are usually those things in our own lives that need the most attention.

The following are some of the things we did which held us together
- Focused on the good things we had in our relationship
- Held on tight to one another when that was all we could do
- Worked on being kind for twenty-four hours a day every day
- Took responsibility for the words that came out of our mouth
- Let go of the idea that either of us would change

- Watched our body language
- Forgave whatever needed forgiving
- Shifted our attitude towards unconditional love and acceptance
- Took care of ourselves and did not wait for someone else to do this for us
- Made every moment count realizing that life was not a dress rehearsal
- Were grateful for the good things in life which included one another

Life was happy! We were laughing again, as if the last thirty years and all the trouble we created on the fast track had never even happened. We hung onto the lessons learned, and let go of the situations that had been our teachers.

People in our lives who have caused us pain have given us the gift of understanding the pain of others going through that same experience. We could now go on being grateful to all the healers, helper, wizards and guides in our lives who helped us through those difficult times.

With our children, now all in their twenties, it is gratifying to see how wise we finally have become in their eyes! Could we have ever thought that this would happen? Our joy has been in realizing that our children are beginning their adult lives with the wisdom and understanding that took us forty years to learn.

They do not want to be co-dependent with anyone. They are free spirited and will maintain their independence. They take better care of themselves than most of us ever did at their age. And they sure do know how to have fun! We as a generation have taught them well, as we have come to learn the same lessons at the same time.

I spend a lot of time in the company of young adults. They are wise beyond their years. All we have to do is listen to them to know this, but they won't talk if they think they will be judged for what they say.

During the past twenty years our children have been taught many skills. I truly believe that part of their wisdom has come out of all the drug abuse prevention education. I've been teaching this and learning this information right along with them. We have helped these young people understand the process of cycle breaking in their lives with peace making skills, positive choices and healthy detachment from the things they cannot change.

If young people know their choices and what to expect in their relationships, as a result of those choices, then they are several steps ahead of their parents. The drug abuse prevention information that they were given contained much more than just the effects of chemicals on their body. They were taught that chemical abuse is a disease that messes up healthy relationships. "Get a life!" they learned to say to their co-dependent parent, or friend, who could not let go of their control issues and live their own life. Many young people today are able to recognize the dysfunctions within their families and have tried to protect themselves from them.

It is a tough lesson for anyone to understand, especially, if they are living in the middle of the craziness and everything "messed up" seems normal.

John Bradshaw writes in his book, *Bradshaw: On The Family,* "If you don't give it back, you will pass it on." Young people understand these things, even if they have not yet found their inner strength to act on what they know to be true. I have great faith that they too will find their healers, helpers, wizards and guides along their path through life when it becomes important to them. For now we can just hope they do not hurt themselves while they learn their lessons.

At Thanksgiving I sent our children the following poem telling them that, as time has passed, we only remember the good times. Again this reflects the wonderful power of the mind and spirit to stay positive.

When You Thought I Wasn't Looking

When you thought I wasn't looking, I saw you hang my first painting on the refrigerator, and I wanted to paint another one.

When you thought I wasn't looking, I saw you feed a stray cat, and I thought it was good to be kind to animals.

When you thought I wasn't looking, I saw you make my favorite cake just for me, and I knew that little things are special things.

When you thought I wasn't looking, I heard you say a prayer, and I believed there is a God I could always talk to.

When you thought I wasn't looking, I felt you kiss me good night, and I felt loved.

When you thought I wasn't looking, I saw tears come from your eyes, and I learned that sometimes things hurt, but it's all right to cry.

When you thought I wasn't looking, I saw that you cared, and I wanted to be everything that I could be.

When you thought I wasn't looking, I looked…and wanted to say thanks for all the things I saw, when you thought I wasn't looking.

Author Unknown

Most of us would love to have the chance to rewrite our past, but in reality I would not have known how to do it any differently. We just did not know that we had choices for these experiences to be anything except what they were at the time.

They were the lessons in my life that I needed to learn in order to bring me to this place in time. It has been my many healers, helpers, wizards and guides that helped me separate out my pain and see the good things around me that we, as a married couple all these years, also created.

We were grateful and happy that we had chosen to weather the storms and not let all the "stuff" separate us. They were good choices. My husband and I are the best of friends and we both know that. I think we always knew it even though we got side tracked for a while, each moving in our own direction. Fortunately for us, that direction went full circle and ended up where it began!

A Friend

Someone whom you can share your inner feelings with…knowing you won't be judged or rejected.

Someone who gives freely… without expectation or motivation.

Someone who lets you be who you are…if you want to change, it's up to you.

Someone who is there when you're hurting… offering true tenderness.

Someone who sees your beauty… your true beauty.

Someone who gives you space when it's needed.. without hesitation.

Someone who listens…
to what you're really saying.

Someone who will consider your different beliefs …
without judgment.

Someone who you always feel close to …
even when they are far away.

Someone who is comfortable to be with…
anytime, anywhere, doing anything.

A friend is a special gift…
to be cherished forever.

Author Unknown

CHAPTER SEVENTEEN

Everything In Its Right Time: Understanding My Sixth Sense

About a year after I began Chiropractic care, I had one more dream. Actually, it was two dreams, backed up to one another on the same morning. Both included wild animals.

In the first one a raccoon came out to me from behind the fence in front of my neighbors house in New York to let me know that it had gently cornered a small animal that was uninjured, but frightened. The raccoon wanted me to rescue it and made sure that I knew it did not want to hurt anyone. The little animal was safe and really did not need my help. It could find its way back home without me!

The second dream was much more powerful. I was again in New York where I grew up as a child, as I dreamt.

I was hearing noises upstairs in the attic off of one of the bedrooms. I went up there and found a wild animal had eaten its way through the wall with its very large ferocious teeth.

I called it a ferret, but it had a very long snout and was showing me many fangs, as it pushed its way through the wall out of the attic. I could hear it snarling, as it poked through the wallpaper close to the ceiling. It suddenly lost its footing and support from behind the wallpaper and fell crashing to the floor at my feet.

I had a heavy shirt in my hand and used it to
muzzle the animal's mouth holding its teeth tightly
together. I was not frightened. I felt very strong and
determined. I felt victorious and called downstairs
to tell someone to contact the animal catcher at the
pound. I felt very secure and safe.

What foe had I finally captured? Was it those frightening
secrets of my life, my feelings of abandonment or sadness for
all the incongruities of love and hate in my life? Was it the
helplessness I felt when I came to realize that I could not have
protected anyone else in this world from the physical and
emotional abuse done to them. Or was it the secrets I kept
that prevented me from being myself and seeing my own
reality: a reality that I was only human and could only be
who I was and not what the world thought I should be. All I
knew was that they were now gone, captured and taken
away.

When I was first married, I had told my husband that I
could never imagine how it would have felt to be abused in
any way as a child. Fifteen years into my marriage I knew
exactly how it felt, not through anyone's fault. I just knew. I
had worked with enough abused children and adults by that
time and I felt their pain. I did not know how to detach
myself from their stories and experiences and throughout the
years I had heard many stories.

**No one hurts anyone on purpose. We just do it
when we reach that point in our lives when
nothing else matters, but our survival.**

Admitting that abuse was done to you, by whomever, or whatever, as an organizational system, does not
make you damaged merchandise. It is in the revelation
of our secrets that we find our personal power which
can bring about change to our lives. It shifts the focus of

the pain and allows us to reclaim who we truly are as the person God created us to be.

As a child, physical and emotional abuse had not been my experience directly, only vicariously, by association with those close to me whom I loved, but could not rescue. I felt so responsible and lived my life that way teaching to those students at the bottom of the class, helping kids to understand their voice and personal power and working extensively in dropout prevention. This also included dropping out of life, as in suicide prevention, or poisoning your life, as in drug abuse.

When my mom got sick with encephalitis I was three years old. I was taken away to my aunt's house for six months. I became the perfect child determined to uphold that perfection, so that no one would get sick or hurt again. Unfortunately, God did not give me the personality for that perfection.

My learning style and my working style always gave out a different impression. My husband married an illusion and proceeded, for too many years to try to make it a reality. My right brain would never let me reach that level of perfection with my attention deficit and my giving, caring heart. My priorities were totally set around the needs of my aging parents, my husband and my children.

So I pretended and compromised who I was for what I thought others expected me to be. Whatever I could do to help others be happy always came first.

I didn't know that I could not make anyone else happy. Each of us have to do that for ourselves from the inside out. I could show them some strategies, but only they could create the self-confidence to see their own value and accept the changes in their lives as they grew in mindbodyspirit.

I gave up myself. As a child, when things got closed in at home, my father, as my protector, in his wisdom knew and encouraged me to escape to the out of doors, to nature or to the beach to find that quiet place to be by myself. Sometimes we hid together, to work on his boat, or identify the stars, after a family picnic on the beach.

> **Control was not a word in his vocabulary. He loved the way my mind worked and was never threatened by anything I ever said to him. That for me is the true meaning of unconditional love. I could always be me in his presence.**

He taught us all to accept our mother in her illness, and to love one another unconditionally. No wonder my dream with his reassurance had such significance to me. It gave me the strength I needed along this journey.

As an enmeshed family, we gave up our identity for the sake of the whole, buried in an illusion that we could control our environment by just being nice and good. When we give up our "self", we never know who we are to be and we go through life on that emotional roller coaster always responding to the needs of those calling out to us.

> **This has been my healing journey back to self. The outside now matches the inside and I no longer need to pretend that I'm fine, fine, fine! I can just be me, how ever I am in the moment!**

I believed that my doctor provided me with that same safety to always be myself. I practiced and practiced being me each visit until I got it perfect, even within the restraints of time. The doctor even asked me once, if I thought I was being a rebel in the way I was thinking, or being. I said, "Oh no! Not at all." He added. "Then you are just being yourself." I quietly said, "Yes!" without any explanation.

My Mask, a poem written by my son, Kevin Synowiec powerfully expresses that honest need to return to self.

My Mask

I wish you could see me.
You say hello here and there,
But you don't see who I really am.
It's not your fault, though.
I put up a defense
To protect myself from harsh words,
To shield me from blinding phrases.

When I witness them, my shield goes up.
I act like someone else.
I've become a master of imitation.
I feel like a fake.
Do you see this smile?
This is my number one disguise.
I have many more.

You see, inside of me,
There is loneliness and pain,
A pain no one knows about.
Possibly the suffering of a lost child.
Maybe, I am whom you see.
That's my best trick...
That's how you're supposed to see me.

Maybe, it is my fault.
Am I just shy? Why?
What's wrong with me?
I feel unfinished,
Broken. Removed.
Are we all in this together?
Do you wear a mask too?

I think someday I will take mine off
Just to see what it's like.
Why am I so nervous though?
I want to take off my mask completely,
But I don't know how.

When I first found Belleruth Naparstek's book, *Your Sixth Sense*, six months ago, I picked it up, looked at it and put it back down. A few months ago I decided to order the book and read it. Everything happens in its right time!

I have spent over fifteen years encouraging individuals, mostly teachers, students and parents, to trust their instincts and believe that what they know in their heart is true. I have often told young people who were having difficulty in school that they have Ph.D.'s in Reading Faces! They liked that! I have known of my well developed sixth sense since I was a little girl. I just didn't know until recently how to put it in neutral! At age nine I remember sitting on the door step with my seven year old sister talking about our grandfather's alcoholism.

My whole family has very highly developed intuitive senses. So do our children. My sisters and I have never kept too many secrets. We could always tell if someone were hiding something! None of us had a chance. We were all very connected, as four sisters and a brother.

We just knew things and saw things that other people often missed. It all seemed very normal. This was never denied. In fact it was like a game to us and nothing at all unique. It was very well woven into the fabric of our lives.

As a teacher, mother and seminar facilitator I too have "eyes" in the back of my head. It was so natural to encourage others to recognize and affirm these intuitive senses in themselves. My Irish ancestors obtained passage to America in the 1840's because they were teachers. My immediate family, back three generations, have done extensive recovery work on school/church and family issues relating to co-dependency and accommodation.

I have learned that I am not alone in this understanding. The incongruities of love and hate in my life existed as part of the fabric that brought so many of us together, long before any of us were ever able to talk about our common ground - or anything else for that matter. People today are finally able to talk about these issues openly and understand the part of their journey which create the co-dependent behaviors in their lives. These discussions strengthen and affirm their intuitive abilities.

For several years now studies have indicated that a large percentage helping professionals are children of alcoholics. This would make sense since their early training as co-dependents, would create in them the desire to make the world a better place. For many, school was far safer for them than being at home and we all look to perpetuate that place of safety in our lives. This also explains their powerful intuitive ability which makes them good at what they do.

On the other hand, until these issues are identified and understood, many will unconsciously continue to surround themselves with the same discomfort of their childhood. If they try to escape, they will find themselves the same situations elsewhere. This was part of the pain I had to walk through as I let go of these controls over me one by one.

On my journey I never doubted anything that happened to me. Some things just defied human logic. I have trusted my intuition and my faith in God and listened carefully for directions.

Recently I told my doctor that I refused to negate anything that has happened to me and he agreed, "You shouldn't." I know that I have always been very hypersensitive to the energy around me. I do not see energy, I feel it. I have often referred to my learning style, as being that of an "intuitive learner."

When I facilitate groups in workshops, I work off the energy in the room and connect with my audience very comfortably. I know how to move them gently through a difficult topic and when to back off and give them a chance to catch up. With certain indicators in my programs, which are not canned speeches, I can tell at which level they are able to process the material that I share with them. I choose to have faith in what I am feeling, trusting and knowing.

This is who I am. This is me being myself. I never give this process a second thought now. In teaching strategies for successful living in dysfunctional environments this confidence becomes very important to affirm what a person says they know they "see." This is all part of letting out the secrets of destruction that everyone knows, but don't talk about within the family system.

> **What I was missing throughout this entire journey and through life, was the realization that I could actually learn to put these intuitive energies in "neutral," as Belleruth Naparstek describes in her book, *Your Sixth Sense*. I did not know how, or even think that I had a choice to do that until I read her book. This knowledge for me was like a special awakening.**

Straight from my heart, for fifteen years I have shared information on family systems, personality types and resiliency skills developed from issues I have come to understand through my own life journey. Why couldn't I detach? This was one of the answers I could not find.

Why did I have to keep running away from that which could not be changed? Why did I feel every three months that I had to get away from what I knew I knew? Is the reason the same for others who also feel "boxed in" in their lives?

In those moments my oldest sister describes me, so accurately, as that of a caged bird, frantically trying to get out. She was not quite sure what I was trying to escape from, but somehow through the years I needed to escape at least every three months. The cage with me and my five children under my wing even has eggs with delicate egg shells on the bottom. Sometimes through life I have had to walk on them very carefully.

When I felt controlled by my world with all its rules and materialism, when I could no longer be myself, I would escape as a bird of the air, as a free spirit, from my bird cage and fly off to Long Island to retreat to a safe place where I could again be myself. With the unconditional love of my parents and my sisters and brother and the connection to self that I felt in the presence of the ocean, I could then return home to Michigan with renewed strength to live in my world of creation. We vacationed out there for years for the same reason. We all call it the "healing place."

My challenge in the last few years was to create that same peacefulness in my life wherever I was to be. It had to become an inner peace, if I were to keep it with me.

Now the nest is empty and the bird cage is gone and that peacefulness within I have found in silence, through this healing journey back to self.

This all makes perfect sense to me now. The questions finally subsided when I realized there was a "switch" I could turn off. It was that part of my journey that taught me to let go, and let go again, of the things I could not control which brought me to this point of faith.

I am also convinced that much of this process has been connected to a my own self-esteem issues. I had lost who I was and did not like who I had become. This affected my health. Getting back to being me also affected my health. It was well worth all the effort.

Many authors suggest that when we die, the one question God will ask us is whether or not we were ourselves. I would like to be able to answer, as Leo Booth suggests, "Yes, in Your image."

My honesty and straight forwardness with my doctor was very much part of my healing relationship. From within I became centered and prayed, connecting my mind with the healing intention of my doctor and with that of the Master Mind. With the inner peacefulness of that moment, I could feel the healing taking place within me.

I know now why so many of my friends spoke so highly of their chiropractors. It is their healing touch with pure intentionality that elicit these emotional responses connected to self, trapped deeply within our cells. I became a full participant in faith and trust of the unknown. It is difficult sometimes to accept the kindness and unconditional love from another human being who may know what is best for us even when we feel captured by our pain.

> **Attachment is the great fabricator of illusions; reality can be attained only by someone who is detached.**
>
> **Simond Weil**

Throughout beginning of this healing journey, I had such an attachment to the outcome. I had to learn to give up the control that this attachment created, in order for me to keep it from affecting the process of healing. It took so long because I could not let go of it! This was an uphill climb for me. I just did not know what I did not know.

A system that holds someone in bondage makes them feel obligated. They feel trapped. When they are given the chance to understand and therefore choose their own program for a healthy lifestyle, they have ownership of it and personal responsibility for its outcome. They will then become a full participant in their own journey towards wholeness in mindbodyspirit.

I feared that the pain would overwhelm me and that I could not go through it. I had to tell myself that I was complete in that pain. I embraced it; I moved forward, as I was able to. In faith I believed that I would have the strength to endure it - in God's time and not my time. As in the peeling of an onion, layer by layer, there were many tears. I grew, as I let the tears come with someone I could trust. This helped to get the pain from inside of me to out there for God to take away.   Our daughter, Christine Synowiec, expresses this so well in her poem.

The Light That Shines Ahead

Lord, I need you to walk beside me.
Please take my hand with dignity.
Walk with me to where I must go
On the stairs to reality.

I need you now more than ever,
To clear my mind of all I fear.
I need your hug to warm my heart,
And your hand to wipe my tears.

I see the light beyond my years,
That Lord you guide me to.
I see my future within my reach,
But I must not go without you.

Lord, all this time,
I have stepped toward the light.
I never hide within a shadow,
Nor have I given up without a fight.

I learn from all I do,
And teach with all I know.
My Lord I fear that someday,
The light to guide me will not glow.

The Lord replied: "The light will always glow,
Each day that you do breathe.
You must not fear what lies ahead,
For strength is all you need.

If the step becomes too tough to climb,
And you reach to take my hand.
I may not be the one beside you,
So you must know when to stand.

When your life seems tough to face,
And out loud my name you call,
That is when I stand behind you,
To catch you when you fall."

©1997 Christine M. Synowiec.   Used with permission.

My Spirit Guide, the God within me, held me together and was ready to "catch me," if I fell. But I did not fall. My faith and trust in a higher purpose leading to self-discovery kept me coming back for more.

I know without any doubt that my complete surrender to the unfolding mystery is what allowed the process of healing to take place within me. It took me a while to get there.

Belleruth Naparstek in her book *Sixth Sense* describes intuition as "that which brings knowledge to you through normal sensory channels that by all accounts and logic you are not suppose to get because it is about someone else." When your intuitive senses do not allow you to disengage your everyday connection with people, then it is only logical that you would filter who you are through the eyes of others. Consequent to that, you would lose your self-esteem along with your personal identity, as you become what other people say and want you to be. You, somehow, know and comply to their needs before they even ask anything of you.

Your intuitive sense, leads you to behave the way someone else wants you to behave. So the question then becomes:
- Are you being yourself or someone else?
- Do you know who you are without what you do?
- Are you living your own life?
- Are you living someone else's life without any freedom of choice?
- Can you still remember who you are?

Fifteen years ago I walked a similar path and found myself. With all the trauma and losses that life brought to me in the past few years, I again slipped away. A physical injury to my neck initiated this incredible journey for me, this journey back to self.

I really thought I knew who I was when I began. It was an illusion that kept me connected. It is now my reality that gives me my hope.

As the pressure on my nerves was released within the vertebrae of my neck, my cells remembered those years of my past. I was asked to revisit that place again. I trusted the process, but not without kicking and screaming on the inside. It was not that I kicked and screamed, but rather, experienced the reality of the turmoil within me. It is gone now and that feels good.

This was my experience. Each of us will have our own journey with our own individual circumstances and experiences. It has been a challenging commitment. I had to go through this process at every level of mind, body and spirit to understand it. With honesty and unconditional love from all my healers, helpers, wizards and guides, and with enormous amount of gratitude for their love and support of me, I feel like someone I was long ago.

I am like a young woman with a new lease on life with an emerging wisdom and desire to share this knowledge with whomever God sends to me. At the end of Chapter Two I said my prayer:

Dear God, send to me whoever needs what I have to share or whoever has what You know I need. Help me to be open to receive whatever it is that will help me grow and heal. I will also trust that I will know when to speak and when to remain silent, as I reach out to others.

In Chapter Three I entered Chiropractic care with someone very unique. I could not have taken this journey without him. He facilitated the process of my healing his way and taught me things in silence I never knew I needed to learn. My life is changed forever. His life is also changed. It is the way it works!

The following symptoms have now replaced the pain. They have become very much a part of me!
I like me this way.

Symptoms of Inner Peace

- The tendency to think and act without fear
- An ability to enjoy each moment
- Loss of interest in judging self and others
- Loss of interest in conflict
- Loss of interest in interpreting other's actions
- Loss of the ability to worry (this is a very serious symptom)
- Tendency to let things happen rather than make them happen
- Frequent overwhelming episodes of appreciation
- Increased susceptibility to receive the love offered by others, as well as the uncontrollable urge to extend it

CHAPTER EIGHTEEN

Letting Go So Far That All
That Remains is Faith

My head was so clear for the first time in so many years that I had to forgive myself for not taking the time to take care of me and my health sooner. True healing involves forgiveness. Why did I abandon myself for so long? Why did I have to create the illusion that I was "fine" in order to please others? "Love your neighbor as yourself," but I forgot to love myself first.

I now know the importance of this. You can't give what you do not have. I was not too hard on myself because I truly believe that everything happens in its right time and this was now my time for all this healing to take place. For years I just thought all the resistance I felt was part of the aging process. So I pretended to still have the energy I always had, but it was such an struggle. This cloud of my true reality was always lingering over me to keep me honest.

This has been a time of renewal for me. I have learned so many wonderful lessons. Getting there was not always easy. I believed in the process and now reap the benefits of my commitment.

It has been a time for me to take all the energy that I have expanded in being president CEO of a major corporation - our family of seven for thirty years - and place it where it belonged so long ago. It is a resume that goes beyond any resume. It can be written only from an experiential point of view.

From within I have taken the issue of denied self and moved it through the emptiness and loneliness that came from not having been true to me. You can't give what you don't have until you get it back again. With this emerging wisdom and internal peace and calmness I have been given an expanded opportunity to share the gifts of my experience and knowledge and become the teacher of teachers, along with other healers, helpers, wizards and guides, but now in a broader sense.

By taking all the qualities and attributes learned as a daughter, teacher, wife, mother and friend and I can extend them beyond the limits set by the responsibility of raising a family. I can now go on with my life far richer in mindbodyspirit than I ever believed possible. I am eternally grateful to all those whose presence in my life gave me the encouragement to believe in me.

I have let go of so many of the things that I thought I could, but could not, control. I have let go of my need to help others understand things that would give them more peace and love in their lives. I sit here with a healthy body and a clear head with tons of energy, unafraid, with no place to go - just being! It is an interesting place.

I stay in neutral with my sixth sense, accepting whatever happens and doing whatever comes in front of me to do. I am not depressed. I feel wonderful, "listening with my inner ear," as my friend, Burt Dubin, once said to me. I am no longer on an emotional roller coaster. I just am! Wow!

It took sixteen months of mindbodyspirit healing plus a lifetime to understand that Faith is letting go so far that all that remains is Faith.

The Journey Within

I was told the patient does their own healing.
    I felt my dependency on the facilitator of that
    process.
I was told the visits were all very important.
    I submitted to the rules and made them count.

I was told the muscles would hurt, as they retrained.
    I exercised others to get them all strong.
I was told the cells remember past emotional pain.
    I remembered the pain right along with them.

I was told this old injury would take time to heal.
    Time became only a moment for reflection.
I could feel the gentle touch of the facilitator.
    I prayed for the guidance of his hands.

I could hear the unspoken words calling out to me.
    I said what could not remain unspoken.
I heard the cries for help around me.
    I cried right along with them.

I could feel the safety created by non-judgment.
    I took a chance to be myself.
I felt the resistance to my honesty and sincerity.
    I became more honest and shared my story.

I wanted it done my way in my time.
    I knew it could only be done in God's time.
I heard more cries for help and prayed.
    I cried again right along with them.

I felt the rush of the outside world.
    I remained quiet in my safe haven.
I fired my Guide and saw an unhappy face.
    I said I was sorry and It returned with a smile.

I heard my heart call out the questions.
  I heard my soul release the answers.
I held back my fear to speak my truth.
  I felt my neck and back fall apart.

I tried again to speak my peace.
  My headaches took over all of my body.
I felt trapped, obligated and in bondage.
  I felt the release of my loving energy.

He worked on the surface of my back and my neck.
  My wounds healed deeply from the inside out.
I wanted to be in control of the process.
  My Spirit taught me that I could let go.

I trusted the doctor with love and respect.
  The love I got back I transferred to my family.
I felt craving to fill the emptiness of my losses.
  I replenished the hollows with unconditional love.

I prayed for the common good of my mindbodyspirit.
  I became peaceful and calm within.
I felt I was taken apart in pieces.
  I was put back together to fulfill my mission.

My gratitude overflows my sense of peacefulness.
  I glow with the Spirit of love in my heart.
I let go and let go of my attachment to the outcome
  Until all that remained was my Faith in my God.

Glossary of Terms

Abuse: to misuse; abuse of the body with self-defeating behaviors; use and abuse of toxins, chemicals; to address another in rude language, or impose or cause physical harm on another; to withhold important information

Accountability: to be personally responsible for an outcome

Action steps: guidelines that lead towards the achievement of specific predetermined goals

Activator: a rubber tipped instrument that delivers a controlled, light and fast thrust of pressure, used instead of the hand, to manipulate the vertebrae

Activator Methods Chiropractic Technique: to utilize a system of body mechanics, neurological reflexes and leg length test to check overall spinal balance and to help locate the misalignments in the spinal column

Acute: comes on quickly with severe symptoms for a short amount of time, not chronic

ADHD: (Attention Deficit Hyperactive Disorder) characterized by high levels of physical activity; consistently impulsive, creative; energetic; extremely short attention spans; easily distracted and cannot sit still for any length of time

Addiction: a physical and physiological dependence on a substance or activity that takes over a persons life, affecting personality, work and relationships

Adjustment: to set right; make exact or suitable; align; arrange in place

Adrenaline rush: an hormone produced chemical high followed by an emotionally depressed low; the roller coaster effect of emotional high's and low's

Alexander Technique: places an emphasis on good posture; gently corrects harmful tensions within the body by increased awareness of balance and movement; helps overcome slouching, hunching over, sitting and twisting the spine and other common posture difficulties

Allergy: an abnormal reaction of the immune system to substances that do not cause symptoms in the majority of people.

Anatomy: the structure, or the study of the structure of the body and the relationship of its parts to one another. Combined with physiology it forms the foundation for conventional medicine

Aneurysm: a saclike enlargement of a blood vessel caused by a weakening of its wall. In the brain it can cause a stroke.

Atrophy: the wasting away, or decrease in size of a body part due to an abnormality, poor nutrition or lack of use, as when a muscle atrophies

Aura: an energy field or magnetic field that exists around every person, plant and animal, indicating the state of health, emotions, mind and spirit; subtle energy

Autonomic nervous system: self-governing or spontaneous motor neurons that convey nerve impulses from the brain and spinal cord (Central Nervous System) to smooth muscle, cardiac muscle or glands

Balance: to bring to equilibrium; adjust; to work in harmony

Bed of nails: Chemicals such as alcohol, drugs, certain medicines and caffeine that can affect the natural balance of the human body when used improperly

Biopsy: removal of tissue or other material from the living body for examination in a lab

Blockage: an obstacle, obstruction, preventing a even flow of fluids

Body language: a true communication without words that the body expresses through position and movement

Bodywork: manipulation by the hands to release tension

Breathing: the process of taking air in and out from the lungs; a life force; power; to inhale and exhale air from the lungs; live; pause; rest; to take a breather

Bronchial asthma: allergic reaction usually characterized by smooth muscle spasms in bronchi causing wheezing and difficulty breathing

Bronchitis: inflammation of the bronchi branches of the respiratory passageway within the lungs

Bursa: a sac, or pouch, of synovial fluid located at friction points, as found around joints

Calcification: hardening deposits of calcium around joints or vertebrae

Carbon monoxide poisoning: lack of adequate oxygen at the tissue level due to increased levels of carbon monoxide in the blood.

Cause: that which produces an effect such as the misalignment or malfunction of a body part to bring about disease

Cell: the smallest structural and functional unit of all organisms capable of performing all the activities vital to life

Cell Memory: the ability of a cell to remember events of the past through genetic coding; memory that lives on in the cells of the body, encoded in its physiology

Centering: bringing a focus to one point, the center and midpoint of anything; point to which, and from which things move or are drawn; to become centered

Central Nervous System: that part of the nervous system that consists of the brain and spinal cord; receives and analyses sensory data and directs a response to the body

Cerebellum: the portion of the brain that is concerned with coordination of movements

Chakra: seven energy centers of the body that absorb and emit the life force; energy flows within the body through channels called "meridians" and these seven main energy centers that align down the spine.

Chi: life force of the body which circulates through its meridians or channels

Chiropractic: derived from the ancient Greek word "Cheiro" meaning hand and "Praktikos" meaning doing; a doctor of chiropractic uses the hands to manipulate body parts, mostly the vertebral column, in order to find the cause of discomfort or illness, rather than covering up the symptoms with medication. The practice concerns itself with the relationship between the nervous system and the function or health of the rest of the body and recognizes that only the power that created the body can heal the body.

Chronic: long term or frequently reoccurring, as with pain

Clarity of intention: belief or value, that has high integrity

Clarity of vision: Being able to see ones path without the "fog" createdby emotional resistance

Co-dependency: involves individuals who connect with others in a way that pulls energy from them. These relationships can cause one to lose their identity and self-esteem in that they give up who they are to fulfill the needs of others without choices. They filter who they are and what they do through the "eyes" and approval of other people

Complimentary practitioners: an approach to the patient as a whole in mindbodyspirit stimulating and facilitating the body's self-healing and self-regulating capabilities

Communication: to talk through and discuss issues of importance in a reciprocal way; both parties sharing their thoughts and concerns

Communication deprivation: when information, helpful and necessary for another's peace of mind, is withheld to the point where that individual feels the emptiness of unanswered questions regarding their own well being

Consciousness: a state of wakefulness in which an individual is fully alert, aware and focused

Control issues: the need to dominate, command, direct, check, restrain and limit another; power over another individual

Conventional medicine: symptoms and medical tests used by doctors to access the problem and prescribe treatment. The actual cause may be missed as the symptoms are covered up with medicinal drugs

Correct biology: academically proper anatomical information relating to the structure and function of body parts; especially important in the process of visualization

Cure: to restore to health, to heal, to successfully complete the course of medical treatment; to remedy a successful treatment

Cyst: a sac containing a fluid or other material enclosed in its own distinctive connective tissue wall

Dementia: an organic mental disorder that results in permanent or progressive general loss of intellectual abilities, such as, impairment of memory, judgment and abstract thinking and changes in personality

Dialogue: open discussion on how habitual ideas and emotions can affect a persons mindbodyspirit

Distant intentionality: prayer with the intention to bring good health to another absent from one's presence

Diuretic: an agent which reduces the fluid level of the body; water is a natural diuretic.

Dysfunction: abnormal functioning of a system or organ within the body; the absence of complete normal function to include all components: physical, emotional and spiritual

Dyslexia: impairment of the brain's ability to translate images received from the eyes or ears into understandable language

Dysphagia: difficulty in swallowing

Eczema: a form of dermatitis that causes a reddening, itching inflammation of the skin

Elasticity: the ability of tissue to return to its original shape after contraction or extension

Emotional release: spontaneous release of blocked energy or tension, believed to result from the letting go of physical or emotional trauma

Emotional roller coaster: perpetual movement of one's emotions from a high point to a low point as in the continuous flow of a wave up and down lasting over a period of time

Endorphins: morphine-like substances produced naturally by the body and released into the blood stream after twenty minutes of exercise creating a natural high

Energy: vigor, activity, force; released by the body by the breakdown of nutrient molecules or foods and used in the body's building processes for the construction of bones, growth of hair and nails and the replacement of injured cells

Energy fields: forces of molecular vibration surrounding all living organisms

Entrapment: the sense of being confined, trapped, boxed in with no escape in sight; a feeling of helplessness

Essence: the life force or pure energy of a living plant or animal

Ethereal: light, airy; spiritual, heavenly

Exercise: movement of different body parts for the sake of strengthening them; training with a particular routine to improve ones health and vitality; should include aerobic for heart and lungs; stretching for flexibility; and weight-bearing or resistance training for our bones

Expectation: belief in a particular outcome regardless of the choices or conditions that might influence it

Faith: something to believe in; letting go so far of all the externals so that all that is left is the belief, trust, or understanding that we began with

Fasting: not eating solid food for a specified period of time. Liquids must always be taken and one should not fast longer than forty-eight hours without a doctor's supervision

Fibrocystic disease: a condition in which benign (noncancerous) lumps form in the breast

Follow through: the completion of an activity; to bring closure to a series of actions leading to a particular outcome

Forced meditation/retreat: a time for quiet thought and prayer that comes as a result to an injury or illness when all other options seem out of reach

Forgiveness: to pardon; to let go of issues of anger that rob you of inner peace and the connection to another

Frustration: disappointment when something does not meet a preconceived expectation

Goal setting: preparing strategies for a particular outcome, as a result of planned efforts to reach a specific end or result

Going within: becoming centered and quiet, clearing the mind of its clutter and focusing on the energy of thought, emotion and spirit that arises from inside our body; to listen in silence

Guided imagery: visualization used to create mental movies with positive images of health and wholeness in the mind that help to relax the body and reprogram the mind to promote healing and bring peace and harmony within.

Healing: the process of formulating positive cellular relationships; the emergence of right relationship at or among any one or more levels of the human experience

Healing crisis: a temporary relapse of health, as a healing or treatment process takes effect in the body

Heart of service: connects one to their purpose and mission in life; the reason they believe they are put on this earth.

Heart palpitations: a fluttering or irregular rhythm in the heart muscle

Holistic: an approach to treatment in which the health and well being of the whole person is considered, rather than just specific symptoms

Homeostasis: a constant internal environment within the body that is maintained separate from any external changes that might be occurring

Hormone replacement therapy: the use of synthetic or natural hormones during peri-menopause and menopause while the body source of estrogen and progesterone is transferred from the ovaries to the other cells of the body, such as the adrenal glands, skin, muscles, brain, the

penal gland, hair follicles and body fat. The female body is capable of
making these adjustments depending on the woman's lifestyle and diet.

Hot flashes: the dilation of blood vessels in an attempt to reset the body's
core temperature. They begin as a feeling of warmth at the waist
which creeps up over the chest, back, neck, face and scalp and usually
end with the break out of a sweat.

Hydrotherapy: water used at different temperatures and pressures; Hot
water relaxes improving circulation; cold water constricts blood flow
to reduce swelling and inflammation

Interdependence: joining with one another in mutually enhancing ways

Interference: a disruption in the transmission of nerve impulses through
the spinal cord due to the loss of normal motion or position of the
twenty-four moving bones of the spinal column

Intuition: perception of truths, facts without reasoning; the language of
the soul; the voice inside you that just knows things without explanation

Isometrics: a form of exercise specifically designed to strengthen certain
parts of the body

Letting go: releasing the energy that locks us into believing something
will be different from what it is, a release to freedom of thought when
expectations and attitudes are changed towards a person of situation

Limbic System: a system of nerve pathways in the brain concerned with
the expression of instincts, drives and emotions and the formation of
memory patterns. Thoughts and emotions have a direct impact on this
area thereby effecting circulation, digestion and musculoskeletal
balance

Listening in silence: centering oneself and clearing away the noises in our
mind to arrive at a place of quiet where we can hear our internal
messengers without the interference of destructive thoughts

Manipulation: used by chiropractic, osteopathic, and other therapies to
adjust the spine, joints and tissues

Massage: acupressure and trigger point therapy used to reduce stress and
bring relief from muscle strains and stress-induced headaches and a
stiff neck

Master Mind Connection: the focus of one's energy of thought on the
spiritual thoughts and actions of another through prayer and a sense
of spirit, guiding them in the healing process

Meditation: supports the flow of energy through the body as one connects
with self, as well as with God, to empower the natural   processes of
healing and self-actualization

Menopause: a time to prepare for the springtime of the second half of a
woman's life; a time when menstruation, or a woman's monthly
period stops, marking the end of her child bearing years and the
beginning of her emerging wisdom

Metabolism: the sum of all the biochemical reactions that occur within the body; the "metabolic rate" reflects the energy required to keep the body functioning when at rest

Mindbodyspirit: balanced, working together as one for the common good of the whole; interrelated; physical, emotional, spiritual Muscle tone: a sustained, partial contraction of parts of the skeletal muscle in response to the stretch receptors that pull it in the opposite direction

Muscle fatigue: the inability of a muscle to maintain its strength of contraction or tension.

Nerve: a cord like bundle of nerve fibers that branch off from the central nervous system out to the extremities of the body.

Night Sweat: twin of the hot flash that can disrupt one's sleep

Osteopathy: manipulative therapy which treats the body as a complete working system addressing the mechanical problems within the framework, (the structure, muscles, ligaments, and connective tissue) to relieve pain, improve mobility and restore all around good health

Osteoporosis: characterized by decreased bone mass and increased chance of fractures as the level of estrogen decreases with aging

Passive resignation: a belief that things must be as they are.

Peri-menopause: the early years of change before menopause when a woman gradually stops ovulating and her ovaries slow down the production of estrogen and progesterone.

Physiology: study of the functioning and interaction of the physical and chemical processes of cells, tissues and organs

Physiotherapy: treatment of injuries with the use massage and manipulation to promote healing and well being

Psychoneuroimmunity: the speciality that says that the mind, body and spirit are connected chemically; the interaction between how one thinks, (our mental thoughts) how we feel (our attitudes) and how our immune system functions

Power surges: hot flashes that occur during peri-menopause that seem to have an added strength, as they release heat and perspiration

Referred pain: pain that is felt in a different part of the body from the area that is actually affected. For example, numbness and tingling in the fingers may be caused by a problem within the neck

Reflex: a quick response to a change in the internal or external environment that attempts to restore balance to the system

Relationship: to be connected to self or another for the purpose of completing a goal or outcome

Relaxation therapy: used to relieve stress and tension by systematically relaxing one from head to toe

Reticula Activating System: that part of the brain that only lets in what one focuses on bringing to them only what one wishes to see; for example, red stones or a particular kind of shell on a beach or positive healthy people

Right relationship: the healing of relationship at the emotional level; such as unresolved conflicts with parents; spouse, child

Scoliosis: an abnormal lateral curvature from the normal vertical line of the backbone also known as "curvature of the spine"

Serotonin: neurotransmitter that relays information across nerve endings from one nerve cell to another

Shaman: highly skilled at healing the sick and foretelling the future; they have the ability to enter into a trance or dream state of altered consciousness; They are then able to separate their souls from their bodies and fly to any part of the cosmos to seek the cure or reasons for the illness and thus cure the patient;

Shamanism: A group of highly skilled healers the sick; highly respected throughout history and practiced since prehistoric times

Soft tissue: tissues of the body that include muscles, tendons, ligaments and organs

Somatoemotional release: sacro-occipital release results from gentle manipulations using fine, sensitive touch applied directly, mostly at the cranium and the sacrum; to resolve any compression or distortion of the cranial bones that may be affecting proper function of other parts of the body

Spasm: a sudden, involuntary contraction of large groups of muscles

Spinal Cord: a mass of nerve tissue located in the vertebral canal from which thirty-one pairs of nerves originate

Spirit Guide: meditatively released image from within the subconscious that serves as a close friend; an excellent advisor, spontaneous and aware of feelings and not to be denied or ignored

Stress: an impelling force that creates a "fight or flight" physiological response within the body brought on by any stimulus that produces an imbalance in the internal environment; in time this excessive adrenaline depletes the body of its much needed energy

Stressor: a stress that is extreme, unusual or long lasting and triggers the body to adapt again and again

Stretching: a technique used to ease tension in the muscles, tendons and ligaments Subluxation: defective joint movement caused by spinal misalignment which produces nerve interference resulting in tissue and organ dysfunction

Subtle energy: the energy, aura, that surrounds a person through which vital energy is said to flow; relates to the mental emotional and spiritual self which may be addressed in diagnosis and treatment

Success: the achievement of a set goal

Symptom: a sign indicating a change in the health of the body resulting from some underlying cause or malfunction

T'ai chi chu'an: an ancient Chinese system of health maintenance and self-defense that employs a series of slow, relaxing movements in coordination with breath, postural integration and mental imagery

Therapeutic touch: with the intention to heal and bring wholeness to the body a person places their hands on or near a person's body in a systemic way to speed healing during therapeutic touch

Tosin: a substance that is poisonous to the body

Trauma: a physical or emotional injury caused by an external agent or force, such as, a physical blow or emotional shock

Trigger points: secondary points of muscle tension caused by pain from the spine and connected tissues. When pressed upon these feel like hard nodules.

Verbally nonresponsive: listens without any response with words only body language; verbally non-judgmental

Vision: the capacity to believe in what your heart sees that others cannot see

Visualization: a relaxation technique in which one creates your one's picture, movie, atmosphere and environment in their mind

Water: a natural diuretic that helps the body to metabolize and get rid of fat; appetite suppressor, helps maintain good muscle tone and get rid of waste; recommended amount per day is eight, eight ounce glasses of water

Weight-bearing exercises: movements in which stress is put on the bones such as in walking, jogging, stair climbing, dance, weight training, skiing

Whiplash: the sudden over stretching of the muscles and ligaments supporting the neck and spine resulting in possible injury to the soft, pulpy discs between the spinal bones of the vertebrae

Wholeness: dynamic process of being in right relationship at or among any one or more levels of the human experience

Wizard: wise person; magician; a person who can influence events; any mysterious agency of power

Yin/Yang: From the Chinese Philosophy that explains the interdependence of all elements of nature and the importance of these contrasting aspects of the body and mind; to be in balance before health and well being can be achieved. Yin is the female force and Yang is the male.

Yoga: a combination of meditation, deep breathing and physical exercise that enhances muscle and joint flexibility and helps maintain healthy bones

Selected Reading List

Allen, James. *As a Man Thinketh*, New York: Barnes & Noble, Inc., 1992.

Allender, S.J., Rev. Tom. *The God Within*, Phoenix, AZ: MW Publishing, L.L.C., 1996.

Andrews, Ted. *The Healers Manual: A Beginners Guide to Energy Therapies.* St. Paul, MN: Llewellyn Publications, 1997.

Beattie, Melody. *Co-dependent No More: How to Stop Controlling Others and Start Caring for Yourself.* NY: Harper & Row, Publishers, Inc.,1987.

Becker, R.D., Gail L. *Heart Smart: A Plan for Low-Colesterol Living.* New York: Simon and Shuster, Inc., 1987.

Bloomfields, M.D., Harold H., and Peter McWilliams. *How to Heal Depression.* Los Angeles, CA: Prelude Press, 1994.

Borysenko, Ph.D., Joan. *A Woman's Book of Life.* Riverhead, NY: 1996.

Borysenko, Ph.D., Joan. *Fire in the Soul: A New Psychology of Spiritual Optimism.* New York: Warner Books, Inc., 1993.

Borysenko, Ph.D., Joan. *Mending the Body, Mending the Mind.* New York: Warner Books, Inc., 1987.

Booth, Rev. Leo. *The God Game. It's Your Move.* Long Beach, CA: Spiritual Concepts

Booth, Rev. Leo. *Prayers That Empower*, Long Beach, CA: Spiritual Concepts

Don Campbell, Don. *The Mozart Effect: Tapping the Power of Music to Heal the Body, Strengthen the Mind and Unlock the Creative Spirit.* New York: Avan Books, Inc.,1997.

Canfield, Jack and Mark Victor Hansen. *Chicken Soup Series*, Deerfield Park, FL: Health Communications, Inc., 1993-1998.

Canfield, Jack and Mark Victor Hansen. *Dare to Win.* New York: Berkeley Publishing Group, 1996.

Caudill, Margaret. *Managing Your Pain Before It Manages You.* New York: Guilford Press, 1995

Chopra, M.D., Deepak. *Quantum Healing: Exploring the Frontiers of Mind/ Body Medicine.* New York: Bantam Books, 1990.

Chopra, M.D., Deepak. *The Path to Love: Renewing the Power of Spirit in Your Life.* New York: Harmony Books, 1997.

Chopra, M.D., Deepak. *The Seven Spiritual Laws of Success: A Practical Guide to the Fulfillment of Your Dreams.* San Rafael, CA: Amber-Allen Publishing, 1994.

Covey, Stephen R. *Seven Habits of Highly Effective People: Powerful Lessons in Personal Change.* New York: Fireside Book, 1989.

Cowens, Deborah. M.S.N, R.N. *A Gift for Healing: How You Can Use Therapeutic Touch.* New York: Random House, Inc., 1996.

Dossey, M.D., Larry. *Healing Words.* CA: HarperSanFrancisco, 1996.

Dossey, M.D., Larry. *Prayer is Medicine.* San Francisco, CA: HarperSanFrancisco, 1996.

Dyer, Dr. Wayne W. *Your Sacred Self: Making the Decision to Be Free.* New York: Harper Collins Publishers, 1995.

DeMello, Anthony. *Awareness: The Perils and Opportunities of Reality.* New York: Doubleday, 1990.

DeMartini, Dr. John. *Count Your Blessings. The Healing Power of Gratitude and Love.* Rockport, MA: Element Books, Inc. 1997.

Evans, Patricia. *The Verbally Abusive Relationship.* Holbrook, MA: Adams Medical Corporation, 1993.

Finley, Guy. *The Intimate Enemy.* MN: Llewellyn Publications,1997.

Finley, Guy. *The Secret of Letting Go.* MN: Llewellyn Publications, 1990.

Forward, Dr. Susan and Joan Torres. *Men Who Hate Women and the Women Who Love Them: When Loving Hurts and You Don't Know Why.* New York: Bantam Books, 1986.

Freeman, Jill and Larry J. Freeman. *Your Inner Beauty: Discover and Express the True Beauty Hidden Within.* NY: Park Lane Press, 1996.

Gittleman, M.S. CNS., Ann Louise. *Before the Change: Taking Charge of Your Peri-menopause:* New York: Harper Collins. 1996.

Gorden, M.D., James S. *Manifesto for a New Medicine: Your Guide for Healing Partnerships and the Wise Use of Alternative Therapies.* New York: Addison-Wesley Publishing Co. Inc., 1996.

Guiley, Rosemary Ellen. *The Miracle of Prayer.* N.Y: Pocket Book, 1995.

Hammerschlag, M.D., Carl. *The Dancing Healers.* CA: HarperSanFrancisco, 1990.

Hammerschlag, M.D., Carl. *Theft of the Spirit,* New York: Fireside, RGA Publishing Group, 1992.

Hay, Louise L. *You Can Heal Your Life.* Carlsbad, CO: Hay House, 1988.

Harp, David. *The New Three Minute Meditator.* Oakland, CA: New Harbinger Publications, 1990.

Inlander, Charles B. and Ed Weiner. *Take This Book to the Hospital With You.* New York: People's Medical Society, Wings Books, 1991.

Jacobs, M.D., MPH, Jennifer, Editor. *The Encyclopedia of Alternative Medicine: Endorsed by the American Holistic Health Association.* Boston, MA: Journey Editions, 1997.

Kubler-Ross, Elizabeth. *On Death and Dying,* New York: Macmillan Publishing Co., Inc. 1969.

Kroeger, Otto and Janet M. Thuesen. *Type Talk: the Sixteen Personality Types That Determine How We Live, Love and Work.* NY: Dell Publishing, 1988.

Margen, Sheldon, M.D. *The Wellness Encyclopedia of Food and Nutrition.* New York: Random House, 1992.

Mike, John, M.D. *Brilliant Babies, Powerful Adults: Awaken the Genius Within.* FL: Satori Press International, 1997.

Millman, Dan. *The Laws of Spirit: Simple, Powerful Truths for Making Life Work.* Tiburon, CA: Linda and Hal Kramer Publishers:1995.

Moyers, Bill. *Healing the Mind*. New York: Doubleday 1995.

Munsch, Robert. *Love You Forever*. Ontario, Canada: 55th Printing, 1997.

Myss, Ph.D., Carolyn. *The Anatomy of the Spirit*. Harmony Books, 1996.

Myss, Ph.D., Carolyn.*Why People Don't Heal and How They Can*. Harmony Books, 1997.

Naparstek, Belleruth. *Your Sixth Sense: Activating Your Psychic Potential*. New York: Harper Collins Publishers, 1997.

Northrup, M.D., Christiane.*Women's Bodies, Women's Wisdom*. New York: Bantam Revised Edition, 1998.

Norwood, Robin.*Women Who Loved Too Much: When You Keep Wishing And Hoping He'll Change*. New York: Pocket Books, 1985.

Oliver, Ph.D., Rose and Frances A Bock, Ph.D. *Coping with Alzheimer's: A Caregiver's Emotional Survival Guide*. New York: Dodd, Mead and Company, 1987.

Pearsall, Ph.D., Paul. *The Heart's Code: Tapping the Wisdom and Power of Our Heart Energy*. New York: Bantam Doubleday Del Publishing Group, Inc. 1998.

Phillips, Vicki. *Empowering Discipline: The Approach That Works with At-Risk Students*. Carmel Valley, CA: Personal Development Publications,1998.

Powell, S.J., John. *Unconditional Love*. Texas: Argus Communications. One DLM, 1978.

Quinn, Janet, Ph.D. *Therapeutic Touch: A Home Study Course for Family Caregivers*. Videotape. New York: National League for Nursing. 1996.

Redfield, James. *The Celestine Prophecy: An Adventure*. New York: Warner Books, Inc., 1993.

Redfield, James. *The Tenth Insight*. New York: Warner Books, Inc., 1995.

Sarno, John E., M.D. *Mind Over Back Pain*. New York: Berkeley Publishing Group 1986.

Sarno, John E., M.D. *Healing Back Pain: The Mind-Body Connection*. New York: Warner Books, Inc. 1991.

Shealy, M.D. Ph.D.., Norman C. and Richard Thomas. *The Complete Family Guide to Alternative Medicine: An Illustrated Encyclopedia of Natural Healing*. Rockport, MA: Element Books, Inc., 1996.

Sheehy, Gale. *The Silent Passage*. New York: Random House, Inc.,1991.

Siegel, M.D., Bernie S. *How to Live Between Office Visits*. New York: Harper Collins 1995.

Siegel, M.D., Bernie S. *Love, Medicine & Miracles*. New York: Harper and Row, Publishers, Inc., 1986.

Simon, Sidney B. *Caring, Feeling, Touching*, MA: Sidney Simon Publications, 1976.

Simon, Sidney B. and Suzanne Simon. *Forgiveness: How to Make Peace With Your Past and Get on With Your Life*. New York: Warner Books, Inc.,1988.

Simon, Sidney B. *Getting Unstuck: Breaking Through the Barriers to Change.* New York: Warner Books, Inc., 1990.

Simonton, O. Carl, and Ried Henson.*The Healing Journey.* New York: Bantam Books,1992.

Smith, Ann W. *Grandchildren of Alcoholics*: Florida: Health Communications, Inc. 1988.

Subby, Robert. *Lost in the Shuffle: The Co-dependent Reality..* Deerfield Beach, Florida: Health Communications, Inc. 1987.

Sun Bear, Wind, W. and Crysalis Mulligan. *Dancing with the Wheel. The Medicine Wheel Workbook.* New York: Fireside Book. Simon & Shuster, 1991.

Synowiec, M.S., Bertie Ryan. *Does Anyone Hear Our Cries For Help? Strategies for Successful Living in Difficult Situations.* Grosse Ile, MI: Positive Support Seminars and Publications, 1995.

Synowiec, M.S., Bertie Ryan. *Quick and Easy Self-Esteem Builders.*Grosse Ile, MI: Positive Support Seminars and Publications, 1990.

Tanner III, Ph.D., W.C. "Tres" and Susan Tanner, M.S. *Enjoy the Journey Along Your Marriage Highway.* San Diego, CA: The Family Connection,1997.

Tenney, M.H. Louise and Deborah Lee. *Today's Herbal Health for Women: The Modern Woman's Natural Health Guide.* Pleasant Grove, UT: Woodland Publishing, 1996.

Weed, Susun S. *The Menopausal Years: The Wise Woman Way.* Woodstock, New York: Ash Tree Publishing, 1992.

Weil, M.D., Andrew. *Eight Days to Optimum Health.* New York: Alfred A Knopf Inc.,1998.

Weil, M.D., Andrew. *Spontaneous Healing- How to Discover and Enhance Your Body's Natural Ability to Maintain and Heal Itself.* Ballantine Books by arrangement with A. Knopf 1995.

Whitfield, Charles. *Healing the Child Within: Discovery and Recovery for Adult Children of Dysfunctional Families.* Deerfield Beach, FL: Health Communications, Inc. 1987.

Wholey, Dennis. *The Courage to Change.* Boston, MA: Houghton Miffin Company, 1984.

Woititz, Janet Geringer. *Adult Children of Alcoholics,* Florida: Health Communications, Inc.,1983.

Woodham, Ann and Dr. David Peters. *Encyclopedia of Healing Therapies,* Dorling Kindersley Limited, 1997.

Vitale, Barbara Meister. *Free Flight: Celebrating Your Right Brain.* Torrance CA: Winch Associates/Jalmar Press, 1984.

Zimmer, Judith. *Weight Watchers Complete Exercise Book.* New York: Macmillan General Reference, 1995.

Book Order Form

❏ **Telephone orders:**
Call Toll Free: 1-800-676-3806

❏ **E-mail orders:** bertie@wdl.net

❏ **Postal Orders:**
Positive Support Seminars,
Bertie Ryan Synowiec,
28641 Elbamar Drive,
Grosse Ile, MI 48138-2013

❏ **Internet: Review this and other books by
Bertie Ryan Synowiec at Bookzone:**
http://www.bookzone.com/bookzone/10000641.html

❏ **Program/Seminar information:** 1-800-676-3806

❏ **Please send me the following books:**

_____

_____

_____

Name _____

Address _____

City _____ State ____ Zip _____

❏ **Sales tax: Add 6% sales tax for Michigan**

❏ **Shipping: $3.25**

❏ **Quantity discounts available**

❏ **Payment enclosed.**